Practice Manual for
Microvascular Surgery

Practice Manual for Microvascular Surgery

ROBERT D. ACLAND, M.D., F.R.C.S.

Professor and Director
Center for Microsurgical Studies
Division of Plastic and Reconstructive Surgery
Department of Surgery
University of Louisville
Louisville, Kentucky

with 158 illustrations
illustrated by Nadine Sokol

Second Edition

The C. V. Mosby Company

ST. LOUIS • WASHINGTON, D.C. • TORONTO   1989

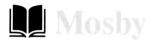

Editor: Eugenia A. Klein
Editorial Assistant: Robin Sutter
Project Manager: Mark Spann
Design: Rey Umali

Second edition

Previous edition copyrighted 1980

Printed in the United States of America

The C. V. Mosby Company
11830 Westline Industrial Drive, St. Louis, Missouri 63146

Library of Congress Cataloging-in-Publication Data

Acland, Robert D.
    Practice manual for microvascular surgery / Robert D. Acland;
illustrated by Nadine Sokol.—2nd ed.
        p.   cm.
    Rev. ed. of: Microsurgery practice manual / Robert D. Acland.
1980.
    Includes index.
    ISBN 0-8016-0006-5
    1. Microsurgery—Techniques.   I. Acland, Robert D.   Microsurgery
practice manual.   II. Title
    [DNLM: 1. Microsurgery—laboratory manuals.   WO 512 A184m]
RD33.6.A25 1988
617'.413059—dc19
DNLM/DLC
for Library of Congress   88-8320
                                                                        CIP
    C/GW/W 9 8 7 6 5 4 3 2 1

To my friend Frank Allen, a dedicated teacher
of microsurgery

Preface

This manual is a practical step-by-step guide for the surgeon who intends to acquire a high level of basic skill in microvascular surgery by means of laboratory practice. Originally written for the use of trainees in the University of Louisville Microsurgery Laboratory, it has now been expanded and largely rewritten to meet a wider need. The second edition has been vigorously revised, with new illustrations throughout and new chapters on end-to-side continuous, and one-way-up anastomosis.

Many of the important principles and details of microsurgical technique described here are derived from the work and teachings of my fellow workers in the microsurgical field. In particular I wish to acknowledge my debts to Drs. Julius Jacobsen III, Harry J. Buncke, John R. Cobbett, Takao Harashina and Daniel Man.

I am also much indebted to the many trainees of the Center for Microsurgical Studies at the University of Louisville. Their successes and difficulties were the chief stimulus to the writing of this manual. Directly or indirectly they have provided many of the practical insights that are included here.

I have had the good fortune to be the Director of the Louisville Laboratory since its establishment in 1975. The Laboratory was set up as a center for microsurgical training and research with the professional and financial support of Drs. Harold E. Kleinert, Joseph E. Kutz, and Graham D. Lister, and with the advice and encouragement of Dr. Hiram C.

Polk, Jr., Chairman of the Department of Surgery at the University of Louisville. I am indebted to them all. I am most grateful to my secretary, Lynn Newton, for her work in the preparation of the manuscript.

Robert D. Acland

Contents

Introduction

The purpose of this manual is to help you learn the basic techniques of microvascular surgery. Even if you have already done a little of this work, I would respectfully suggest that you begin at the beginning. Many of the common sources of difficulty are covered in the early sections of the manual.

PRACTICE TIME

If you intend to learn as well and as rapidly as possible, do your utmost to set aside at least one uninterrupted week when you will have no commitments other than to be in the laboratory undisturbed. Learning microsurgery will initially make great demands on you. You should try to sleep well, be at peace with the world, and disengage yourself from the demands of the clock and the telephone. It is unrealistic to expect to learn well during hasty and sporadic sessions snatched out of a busy schedule when other responsibilities are clamoring for your attention.

At the onset, you may find it hard to believe that you will ever reach the stage where microvascular anastomosis becomes easy. When you do reach it, it will be because you have studied the apparent difficulties systematically and have learned to overcome them for yourself.

AVOIDING DESPERATION

There is no single stroke of magic in mastering microsurgical technique. Rather, the process involves learning to put together a large number of different points of detail, each one of which is simple and readily understood. Almost everyone finds that the first day or two are somewhat frustrating. Do not be discouraged by this. Often it is when you seem to be progressing most slowly that you are in fact learning most. After one or two days you will reach a point where you suddenly seem to "get it all together" and the work will become a pleasure.

Remember that you are learning a technique in which the margin for error is measured in thousandths of an inch. Do not be alarmed by this. Accept it calmly, and it will help you to master each step thoroughly before progressing to the next. If you press on too fast, your learning will be incomplete. It is better to progress more slowly and to learn solidly.

DO NOT STRUGGLE WITH DIFFICULTIES—A FUNDAMENTAL RULE

If something is wrong, do not struggle on. If you do, one difficulty will lead to another, and dificulties lead to disaster. When a difficulty is perceived, *stop*. Whatever the difficulty—unwanted movement, an uncomfortable position, an eyepiece out of focus, a blood-stained field, a blunt needle, forceps that will not grip, untidy vessel ends, or a thread that you cannot pick up—do something about it before you go further. Either figure out what is wrong and put it right, or ask for advice.

SMOKING, COFFEE, AND OTHER BAD INFLUENCES

Smoking a cigarette will noticeably impair your concentration and performance for about 30 minutes. If you have to smoke at all, do it outside the laboratory. Stick to your normal coffee drinking habits. Admittedly coffee causes a slight tremor, but acute coffee withdrawal causes a worse one.

Two factors that give rise to more tremor than either coffee or smoking are irritation and strenuous manual exertion. Do your utmost to avoid having your practice time clouded by extraneous sources of irritation. In addition, do not allow yourself to become irritated at the difficulties that you face during practice sessions, but accept them as constructive experiences to be studied and overcome.

Strenuous manual exertion such as heavy lifting, playing tennis, or holding on to hip retractors will make it very difficult for you to use your small muscles precisely. Such work leaves a residue of tremor for about 24 hours afterward and should therefore be avoided during the day preceding your start in the laboratory.

Lack of sleep will severely impair your learning performance. If you have been up all night, go and get some sleep.

DURATION OF PRACTICE SESSIONS

Avoid working for too long at a stretch. Your time in the laboratory is valuable and limited, but you will be using it uneconomically if you try to work right through the day without taking breaks. If you work in this way, you will suffer severe impairment of your judgment, your coordination, your ability to learn, and your ability to deal intelligently with difficulties. You should regularly take a break for ten minutes every hour. It is difficult to do this of your own volition, and frequently you will be advised by someone else that you should take a break. When this advice is given, do not resist it. The insistence on continuing when your performance has already fallen off is one of the first signs of impaired judgment. If someone advises you to take a break, take a break.

chapter # 1 Equipment for microsurgical practice

This chapter describes all the equipment you need for the work described in this book. Addresses of supplying companies and catalog numbers of individual instruments can be found at the end of the book.

GET YOUR OWN INSTRUMENTS

The instruments needed for good microsurgical practice are few and simple, but they must be of excellent quality and they must be your own. If you do not yet have a set of good instruments, order them now and wait until they arrive before you start. Pay no attention to the widespread belief that any old, worn out, battered, or obsolete equipment is "good enough for the lab." It isn't.

The instruments described here are used in the Louisville Laboratory. They have been chosen for quality, inexpensiveness (where possible), and simplicity.

SPRING TENSION

Be sure that all the spring-handled instruments you choose have the right spring tension. If the tension is too weak, the tips will come all the way closed the moment you put enough pressure on the instrument to get it settled in your hand. If the tension is too firm, your thumb muscles will become painfully fatigued. To test the spring of an instrument for weakness, pick it up and hold it with just enough force that the tips are 1 to 2 mm apart. Then, maintaining just that force, pronate your forearm completely so that the instrument hangs upside down. If it falls away from your hand, the spring is too weak. To test for excessive firmness, hold the instrument gently closed for 10 minutes. If you feel pain in your thenar muscles, the spring is too strong. Choose only instruments whose spring tension lies between these extremes.

JEWELER'S FORCEPS   Straight fine-pointed no. 3 jeweler's forceps (Fig. 1-1) are used almost continually in the non-dominant hand for tissue handling and suture tying. Their tips must be aligned with a precision of 1/1000 inch, since that is the diameter of 10/0 nylon. When closed with moderate pressure the jaws should meet not only at the tips but also evenly over a length of 3 mm so that thread can be picked up easily. The only jeweler's forceps good enough for microsurgery are those stamped with the trademark of Dumont. Dumont forceps from the recommended supplier are individually refinished under the microscope for microsurgical use.

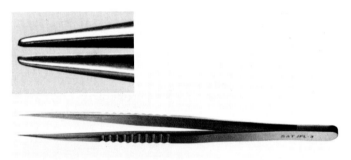

Fig. 1-1

ANGLED JEWELER'S   Angled jeweler's forceps (Fig. 1-2) have a number of
FORCEPS   special uses, including reaching under a vessel, tying

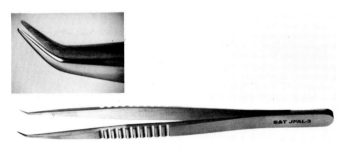

Fig. 1-2

knots, and doing patency tests. They should meet at the tips as exactly as the straight ones should do.

NEEDLEHOLDER

Pick a round-handled needle holder with fine, fully curved jaws and without a lock. Look for an open gap at the point shown by the arrow in Fig. 1-3. If that gap closes right up when the jaws close, your thread will often get trapped there.

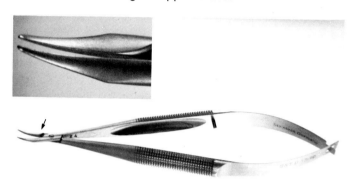

Fig. 1-3

VESSEL DILATOR

A vessel dilator is a modified jeweler's forceps with a slender, smoothly polished, nontapering tip (Fig. 1-4). It is put inside the vessel end and opened a little to produce gentle dilatation. It is also useful as a counterpressor for suturing in confined places.

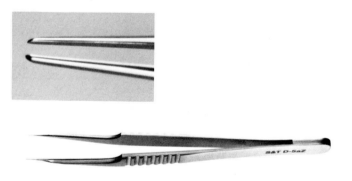

Fig. 1-4

DISSECTING SCISSORS

Dissecting scissors should be spring handled, should have gently curved blades, and should be lightly rounded at the tips (Fig. 1-5). The rounded tips are important. They enable you to dissect very closely

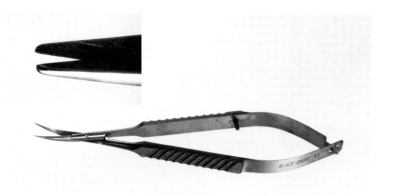

Fig. 1-5

along a vessel without the danger of making a hole in it.

ADVENTITIA SCISSORS For the special task of trimming the adventitia off the vessel end, you need a pair of fine, straight microscissors with very sharp pointed tips (Fig. 1-6).

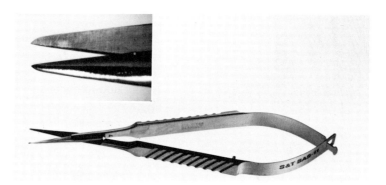

Fig. 1-6

The round-pointed dissecting scissors will not do this fine work properly. Their tips are too bulky for it. Adventitia scissors are also good for stitch-cutting: it does not damage them.

VESSEL CLAMPS The full range of exercises described in this manual calls for the small collection of clamps shown below (Fig. 1-7, *A*). The set includes one comparatively large sliding approximator clamp with built-in suture-holding frame, for beginning anastomosis; a smaller plain approximator clamp for more

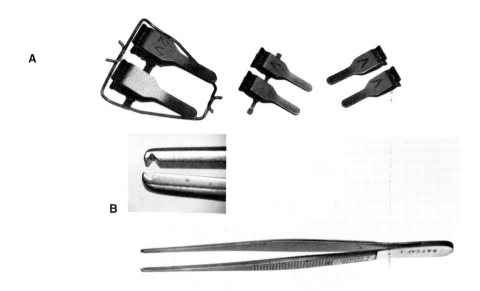

A

B

Fig. 1-7

advanced exercises; and two small single clamps. The clamps have flat gentle jaws. The larger ones, 11 mm in length, have a spring tension that is calibrated to make them almost harmless on vessels between 1.5 and 0.7 mm in diameter. The smaller 8 mm clampshave less closing force and are for vessels 1.0 to 0.4 mm in diameter.

Along with the clamps, you need a clamp-applying forceps Fig. 1-7, *B*—don't use any other instrument than this to apply clamps or take them off.

NONMICROSURGICAL INSTRUMENTS

For the macrosurgical tasks of incision and initial exposure you need a No. 15 scalpel, a pair of fine-toothed forceps, and a small pair of ring-handled scissors.

INSTRUMENT CASE

As soon as you get your instruments you must have a safe case to keep them in. If they are not kept in a good case, they will quickly be damaged. A proper instrument case is quite expensive. It is autoclavable and has a rack with a slot for each instrument. A cigar box will do the job well enough at first. Fill it up with two layers of soft packing material, such as foam rubber, and keep the instruments sandwiched between the two layers so they cannot move around.

INSTRUMENT CARE

Take good care of your instruments and they will last a long time. Make it a rule that their tips will never touch another hard object. Keep them away from heavier instruments, do not pick them up more than one at a time, and avoid putting the tips down on the table. Do not lend them to anyone, ever.

The best way to clean microinstruments is to submerge them completely for 30 minutes in a hemolytic enzyme solution such as Hemosol. This dissolves even the hardest blood clot. Then rinse the instruments in water. Rinse the clamp hinges specially well with a brisk jet of water from a syringe. Then dry the instruments thoroughly before putting them away.

Minor repairs and readjustments can be made to the tips of jeweler's forceps with the aid of a fine pair of flat-jawed pliers, a small white Arkansas oilstone, and some 4/0 jeweler's emery paper. This work needs to be done under the microscope.

MAGNETIZATION

Occasionally instruments become magnetized from contact with a magnetized object, from contact with electrical equipment containing electromagnets, or from being reground. The only cure is an instrument demagnetizer, which is a simple, hollow, electric coil connected to the regular AC supply. Place the instrument inside the coil, switch on the current, slowly withdraw the instrument until it is 2 feet away, then switch off the current. A tape-deck demagnetizer will just suffice for treating instruments, but it is rather weak and must be used very slowly.

BIPOLAR COAGULATOR

The bipolar coagulator is indispensable for high-grade hemostasis. Using it effectively is one of the basic skills you will be learning. A plain single-function bipolar unit is enough, together with a good pair of bipolar forceps. The best bipolar forceps are the inexpensive, semidisposable ones that come with a cord attached.

SUTURE

For suturing, use flat-bodied microvascular needles on 10/0 monofilament nylon. High-grade flat-bodied needles 100 and 75 microns in diameter are now readily available in unsterile "Lab Pack" packages. Use the 100-micron size for basic exercises, 75 micron for advanced exercises. Round-bodied needles, which are very hard to control, are happily almost a thing of the past.

MICROSCOPES

Do not get more microscope than you need. You can learn to do good work by yourself with a simple single-person microscope mounted on a bench stand. If you are setting up a laboratory where instruction will be given by an expert, you need a twin-head microscope; otherwise you don't. Foot-operated remote control for magnification and focusing is a great convenience, but is not truly a necessity. You can learn good technique on a hand-operated microscope.

The microscopes best suited for laboratory work are those made by Zeiss and by Wild. Microscopes of other makes tend to have imperfect optics, which sharply limit the precision of your work at high magnification. Zeiss and Wild optics are exactly comparable, despite what each manufacturer may claim. The illuminators of old Zeiss microscopes tend to be inadequate for work at high power; however, better illuminators can readily be retrofitted. The best focal length for the objective lens for general purposes is 200 mm provided you are of normal height. If you are exceptionally tall, a 300 mm objective will give you a better working position. The best eyepiece magnification is ×12.5. In a microscope having a magnification changer or zoom system of average range, the combination of ×12.5 eyepieces and 200 mm objective gives a magnification range of 4 to 20, which is plenty.

OLD MICROSCOPES   There are old Zeiss microscopes living in retirement in many hospital departments. You may have access to one. You will possibly find the adjustments are stiff, the eyepieces out of alignment, the light source dim, or the wiring faulty. Have a good service technician look the microscope over and give an estimate for overhauling it. It might be the best way to get yourself a good working microscope.

CARE OF THE MICROSCOPE   Each time you use the microscope, clean the outer glass surfaces of the eyepiece and objective lenses with lens tissue. Avoid getting dust inside the microscope, as will happen if it is left standing with the eyepieces or the binocular head removed. If the microscope has to stand unused for long periods, wrap the whole head in a plastic bag.

If you have to move a microscope, do it carefully because this is the time when microscopes are damaged. Remove the microscope head and carry it separately. Do not move a microscope floor stand any distance on its own small wheels. Put it on a cart with large rubber wheels—a four-wheeled tilting oil drum cart is ideal. Do not move a heavy microscope just before a practice session—the exertion will increase your tremor.

FURNITURE   The table or workbench at which you practice should be 30 to 33 inches high. It should be very solid. It is important to be able to sit with your knees under the worktop and your feet planted well in front of you. Therefore avoid a work top that has a drawer or any other obstruction beneath it. If two people are to work together on opposite sides of a table in comfort, the table should be 20 to 24 inches wide.

Your stool should have feet, not wheels. It should be easily adjustable to a comfortable height for operating. A backrest is unnecessary, and arms are a nuisance.

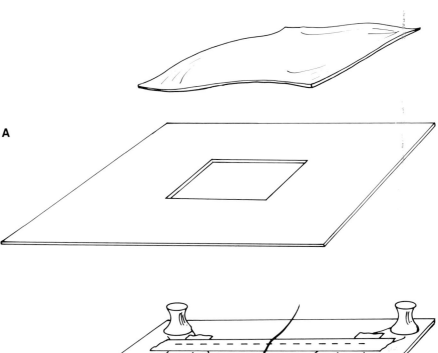

A

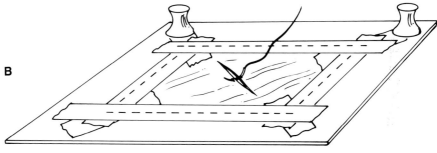

B

Fig. 1-8

GLOVE-RUBBER PRACTICE CARD Your initial suture exercises will be done on a piece of glove rubber stretched out on a practice card. You will need to make one or two of these. Take a 3-inch square piece of strong cardboard and cut out a 1-inch hold in the middle of it (Fig. 1-8, *A*). Take a 2-inch square piece of rubber cut from a surgical glove and stick it centrally on the card with tape. It should be under just enough tension to get the wrinkles out. When in use, the whole practice card is taped to the work top to avoid unwanted movement.

RAT BOARD The rat board should be 12 inches long and 8 inches wide. The best material for a rat board is Homosote, a fiber board lined on both sides with cork, that is used for bulletin boards. It accepts push pins easily and is washable. Avoid the kind that has cork on one side only because it warps too much. The rat board should be equipped with several push pins and two retractors. A good retractor is made from a regular paper clip, reshaped to have a hook at one end and an eye at the other. An elastic band is doubled through the eye (Fig. 1-9). The hook is placed on the wound edge, and the elastic band is stretched out and secured with a push pin.

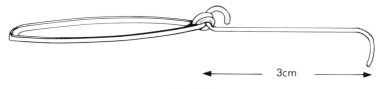

3cm

Fig. 1-9

BACKGROUND MATERIAL

You must have some well-colored, opaque, plastic sheeting to put behind the vessel to provide visual contrast. Deep blue is a very satisfactory color. The best source of blue plastic sheeting is a string of blue, white, and red bunting flags. Either find a suitably decorated service station and speak to the manager or buy a whole string for yourself.

CLIPPERS AND DEPILATOR

It is essential to have the animal clean shaven in the operative area. Rats have very dense fur, so this is not an easy job. You need a good electric clipper with the finest grade cutting head.

SURGICAL SUNDRIES

To fix the rat to the rat board you need 1-inch adhesive tape such as autoclave or masking tape. To keep the wound wet you need a 20 cc syringe with a 25-gauge needle filled with lactated Ringer's solution. To remove excess liquid from the wound have a supply of 4 × 4 surgical sponges. For anesthesia use injectable pentobarbital (Nembutal) diluted 1:10 with distilled water (6 mg per ml). Give this intraperitoneally, first with a 5 cc syringe and subsequently through a scalp vein needle strapped into place (see Fig. 9-2, p. 46). For vasodilatation use 1% plain lidocaine (Xylocaine).

chapter **2** **Essential preparation: getting comfortable and adjusting the microscope**

THE IMPORTANCE OF COMFORT

If you have learned elsewhere in surgical training that you ought to disregard your own comfort, get ready now to learn just the opposite. In microsurgical work, comfort is a precondition of success. Discomfort will steadily erode your ability to concentrate and your willingness to take trouble; it will destroy your skill. Take this opportunity to get into an important and permanent habit, that of making yourself thoroughly comfortable *before you get started.*

Making room for your legs. To do this begin at floor level. Remove all obstacles that stop you putting your feet where they belong—under the table. If the microscope has a foot pedal, get that in place so that one of your feet can be on it all the time. If anything stops your knees from getting right under the table, remove it, or move to a more accomodating table.

How you sit. Having made a space for your legs and feet, consider seriously how you are going to sit. This is fundamental! The way you sit directly affects two vital things: how well you can control the movements of your fingertips and how well you can see down the microscope. To do fine fingertip work without a tremor, you must sit so that your arms rest passively on the table doing nothing. To maintain a stable view down the microscope, you must sit so that your head remains motionless. Keeping your head motionless means keeping your upper body quite still.

How you keep your upper body still is important. The way *not* to do it is to prop yourself up by leaning on your elbows. This is a big mistake in microsurgical work. Leaning on your elbows to stabilize your body makes many of your arm muscles busy and tense, and this immediately produces tremor. Instead of leaning on your elbows you must keep your upper body still by maintaining a perfectly balanced sitting position. It is easy to learn to do this: proceed as follows.

Move back from the table so that no part of you is touching it and let your arms hang down by your side. Plant your feet separately and equally on the floor in front of you and make up your mind to keep them there. With your neck and your back comfortably straight, tilt your body forward and backward a little and find the angle of tilt that you can maintain with the least amount of effort. That is your balanced sitting position. Isn't is surprising how still you can sit?

Lift one of your feet off the floor for a moment. The quick feeling of imbalance this gives you shows at once how important your feet are as stabilizers. Make sure that you keep them on the floor in front of you at all times. If you cross your legs or tuck your feet beneath your seat they cannot act to stabilize your body position. If one of your feet is on the foot pedal of the microscope, that's fine provided it goes on bearing its share of your body weight. Having settled on a good sitting position, move your stool forward until your body just barely touches the edge of the table.

Your next concern is to ensure that your eyes are at the right height in relation to the eyepieces, and that your head and neck are inclined at an angle that you can comfortably sustain. This involves two interrelated

---

adjustments: the height of the stool and the tilt of the microscope head.

THE EXIT PUPIL AND THE OPTICAL AXIS

Here we need a one-page digression on optics. You are about to accomodate your whole big body in relation to two important little features called the exit pupils. These lie in mid-air just a short distance from the surface of each eyepiece. The stream of focused light leaving each eyepiece is a converging cone that reaches a narrowest diameter of about 2 mm, then spreads out again. The narrowest point of this double cone, an imaginary disc, is the exit pupil. It lies about 15 mm out from the eyepiece. If you are to see the whole of the view the microscope offers you, then that bright little disc, the exit pupil, must sit right in the middle of the hole in your iris. If any of it misses the pupil and hits the edge of your iris, a huge crescent of your field of view will be cut off. Since your own pupil, under normal light conditions, is only about 3 mm in diameter, the margin for error in the position of your eyes, and of your head, is tiny.

Besides this the position of your head is restricted further still by another factor. This concerns the direction of your line of sight. If you look into the eyepieces at an angle you can't see anything. To see what is there to be seen, each eye must have its line of sight, or optical axis, in just the same line as the optical axis of the eyepiece. The angle at which the eyepieces point has great power over you. It dictates exactly the direction in which you point your eyes. Not only that: it also has a strong effect on the position of your head. This is because for long-term comfort there is just one good position for your eyes relative to your head: looking straight ahead. Looking up, down, or sideways with your eye muscles quickly makes them tired. Because of this, the angle at which you incline your head must correspond within a few degrees to the angle of inclination of the eyepieces.

When you first look down the microscope you may perceive nothing but large incomplete circles of light that fly in and out of your field of vision rapidly and without control. This happens because your head is moving. As soon as you start to keep your head still in the right position, those circles of light will settle in the center of your field of view and you will start to see something, at least with one eye. (You will only see with both eyes when you have adjusted the distance between the eyepieces. That comes later.)

Enough about optics; let's get back to comfort.

PUTTING THE MICROSCOPE IN POSITION

Your next step is to get the microscope head into its working position and for that you must decide where on the table you are going to work. To decide this, take an instrument in each hand, rest your elbows widely apart on the table, and bring your hands together in front of you. Mark the point on the table where the two instruments meet. This will be your best working spot. Put some small object there that you can focus on. Adjust the tilt of the microscope head so that the eyepieces incline at about 50 degrees to the horizontal. (If you are very short, make the angle about 40 degrees. If you are very tall, make it nearer 60 degrees.) Turn on the microscope light and maneuver the microscope so that its circle of light shines on your chosen working spot. Ignoring comfort for a moment, look down the microscope and adjust its head upward or downward until your small object comes into clear focus. This brings the microscope head to its proper working height and position.

ADJUSTING HEIGHT AND HEAD ANGLE

Now that the microscope is in position, you need to get to where you can see down it in comfort. Three things can be adjusted to achieve this: first, the height of the stool, second, the tilt of your head, and last, if necessary, the tilt of the microscope. (Up and down movement of the eyes relative to the head does not count as an adjustment.)

Holding your head at an angle of upward or downward tilt that lies more or less in the range of comfort, adjust the height of the stool till your eyes are at just the right level to see down the eyepieces. Looking down the microscope with your eyes pointing straight ahead, decide whether your head position is truly comfortable. If it is you are ready to go ahead with eyepiece adjustment (see below).

If your head is inclined too steeply downward or upward for comfort, reduce or increase the angle of inclination of the microscope head accordingly. Having changed the angle of inclination, reposition and refocus the microscope on your working spot. By changing the angle of inclination, you slightly altered the height of the eyepieces. So now readjust your stool height to get your eyes back level with the eyepieces. You may have to repeat this cycle of adjustments more than once to reach your best head position.

Once you have thoughtfully gone through the exercise of getting comfortable a few times, doing it will become a habit every time you sit down to do microsurgical work. Don't proceed with what comes next until you are truly comfortable. You will not be able to think critically about what you are seeing if your eye muscles, your neck, your back, and your rear end are all sending loud messages of complaint to your brain.

You have two final adjustments to make—first, the interpupillary distance, then the individual eyepiece focusing adjustment. Both these adjustments are critical to the quality of your view and the success of your work, so be patient.

ADJUSTING INTERPUPILLARY DISTANCE

While you are adjusting the interpupillary distance, both your eyes need to be looking straight ahead. If you make your eyes converge, as though to see something close, your pupils will move together and you will get the adjustment wrong. So, while making the adjustment, tell yourself firmly that you are looking at something in the far distance.

Take the two halves of the binocular head of the microscope in your two hands and move them as far apart as they will go. Turn the magnification to the lowest setting. Put a very small object in the center of the microscope's field of view. With one eye look down the microscope and adjust the main focus until you can see the object clearly. Then, still keeping your eye fixed on that small object, deliberately back your head away from the eyepiece by 2 or 3 cm. As you do this, the circle of light that you can see will become quite small. Keep your head there and keep that small circle of light in the center of that one eye's field of view. Now slowly bring the two eyepieces together. A second small circle, seen by your other eye, will swim into view. Adjust the eyepieces until the two circles meet and become one circle. Then move your head toward the eyepieces again, and you will see two big exactly corresponding circles of light, one for each eye. You now have a fully stereoscopic view.

EYEGLASSES AND THE MICROSCOPE

Each eyepiece contains its own focusing adjustment that will correct for any degree of near or farsightedness just as well as eyeglasses do. If you wear glasses, you have a decision to make—either to keep them on or to take them off and use the eyepiece focusing adjustment. Which you do depends on the strength of your eyeglass correction. If it is between plus one diopter (farsighted) and minus three diopters (nearsighted) you should take off your glasses and use the eyepiece focusing adjustment as described below. If your correction lies outside that range you should keep your glasses on since without them you would have a hard time seeing small things on the table in front of you when looking away from the microscope. If you are going to keep your glasses on, just set the focusing adjustment on each eyepiece to "0", and then make sure the eyepieces are pushed right down in their seating. Assuming that your eyeglass correction is indeed correct, you are now ready to go to work. If you are in any doubt about the correctness of your correction, go through the eyepiece focus adjustment routine described below.

The eyepiece adjustments do not correct for astigmatism. If you have an astigmatic correction, you must keep your eyeglasses on.

(If you have deep-set eyes or a prominent nasal bridge, your eyeglasses may sit so far from your eyes that you cannot get close enough to the eyepieces to see the full view that is available. If this is a major problem, you may need to consider getting a special pair of glasses for microscope work with small lenses that can sit close to your eyes.)

EYEPIECE FOCUSING ADJUSTMENT

There are two equally strong reasons for having the eyepiece focusing adjustments both set just right. The first is that, for your eyes to give you a perfectly sharp three-dimensional picture, they must both receive an equally well-focused image. This can only be obtained by having both eyepieces properly set. The second reason to have them correctly adjusted is that when they are correctly set, your carefully focused view will stay sharp regardless of any change that you make in the magnification setting of the microscope. This is referred to as having a parafocal view. With the eyepieces wrongly set you lose parafocality: your view goes out of focus each time you change magnification. This becomes a major annoyance. The annoyance is more than doubled when you start working on a two-person microscope.

Use the following dependable routine to arrive at the correct setting. Before and after doing this routine, make sure that both eyepieces are pushed all the way down into their seatings. Imperfect seating leads to an incorrect setting.

Attend first to one eye and then the other. While doing this routine put the other eye out of business by setting the interpupillary distance, temporarily, a long way out of adjustment. (Holding the other eye tightly shut is a bad way to put it out of business. That distorts the shut eye and subsequently blurs its vision.)

Put an extremely small distinct object on the table in

the middle of the field of view. A piece of paper with a speck of dust on it is ideal.

First eye

1. Turn the magnification to the *highest* setting.
2. Using only the main microscope focus control (not the eyepiece adjustment), get the small object into the sharpest possible focus. Now leave the main focus control alone and don't touch it again.
3. Change the magnification to its *lowest* setting. Almost certainly your view will go somewhat out of focus when you do this.
4. Without touching the main focus control, move the eyepiece focusing adjustment until your low-magnification view comes back into perfectly clear focus. That's it for the first eye.

Second eye

5. Still not touching the main focus control, return to high magnification. Your view with your second eye will be sharp.
6. Change the magnification down to low again.
7. Again adjust the eyepiece focus control until the low magnification view with your second eye is perfectly sharp. That's it for the second eye.
8. Finally, reset the interpupillary distance. You now have your microscope fully adjusted and you are ready to go to work.

By patiently attending to the detailed routine described in this chapter you will have gained two basic preconditions of success in microsurgery—physical comfort and a perfect view of what you are about to do. These in turn will go a long way toward ensuring the most important precondition of all—your peace of mind.

If it takes you an hour to get all these adjustments made to your complete satisfaction, do not begrudge the time. Time spent setting yourself up for success is always time well spent.

3 Preliminary suturing exercises

Plan to spend 3 to 6 hours on the basic suturing exercises described in this chapter. Use the glove rubber practice card described in Chapter 1 (p. 12). Part of the purpose of these exercises is to learn basic suture passing and knot tying. An equally important purpose is to introduce you to good hand position and the avoidance of unwanted movement. In addition, you will gain valuable early familiarity with the operating microscope. If you have not already worked through the important routine of getting comfortable and adjusting the microscope as described in Chapter 2, do so right now.

THE AVOIDANCE OF TREMOR

The uncontrolled movements that arise from the intended and unintended actions of your own body are spoken of collectively as *tremor.* Ignore almost all you hear about the prospective microsurgeon's need to avoid specific vices (see introduction). Such tales are irrelevant. Ignore also the notion that a fortunate few are "born with a steady hand." They aren't. Steadiness of hand is achieved by working at it. The prerequisites are a quiet mind, bodily comfort, and a well-supported hand and instrument-holding position.

POSITION OF HANDS

In microsurgery, only the fingertips move. The rest of your hand must rest either directly or indirectly on an immovable surface. If it does not, unwanted movement will make your work impossible.

Start by working in the "writing" position (Fig. 3-1), as this gives more stability than any other. Rest your

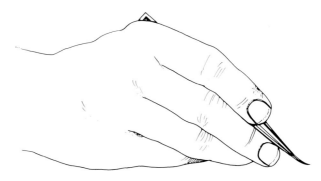

Fig. 3-1

elbow, your wrist, and the ulnar border of your hand on the table. The forearm should be supinated (knuckles away from you) a little so that the weight of the hand is on the ulnar border. Hold the instrument exactly as you hold a pen when writing (Fig. 3-2), using your thumb and index and middle fingers. The middle finger—the lowest member of the three-digit tripod that holds the instrument—should rest firmly on the working surface, either directly or indirectly via the ring finger.

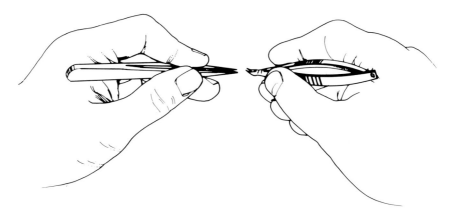

Fig. 3-2

In arranging your three-digit grip on the instrument, bring the thumb and index finger into contact with the underlying middle finger. You will then be able to open and close the instrument with very fine control; any tremor arising from the thumb or index finger will be markedly diminished by their contact with the steady middle finger.

The writing position described is the easiest to start with. Continue using it until the basic manipulations of suturing become easy. Variations and more freehand positions will come later.

Whatever position you are in, you should never have to hold your whole body rigid to perform fine manipulations. If you find you are doing this or that you are holding your breath while you are working, it means that you are struggling to work with your hands in an unsupported position.

Do not put your hands in a position where they bump into the thing you are working on. This produces a lot of unwanted movement—and microsurgery is basically a battle against unwanted movement!

From this point on through the manual the instructions are given on the assumption that you are right-handed. If you are left-handed, kindly make the necessary translations.

CONTROLLING TREMOR WITH DRUGS

In the introduction, in Chapter 2, and in the section just ended, you have read some important advice on self-care, comfort, and hand position. By following this advice almost anyone can overcome the problem of unwanted movement well enough to do excellent microsurgical work. But not quite everyone. If you have an unusually high state of resting muscle tone and if some aspect of the learning situation is making you anxious, you may still have a problem. You may become locked into a vicious cycle in which anxiety and tremor potentiate each other. In such a state you may be unable to achieve the early successes that would give you confidence and steadiness. If this is the case, I advise you as a short-term measure only to take a small dose of the highly effective beta-blocker propranolol (inderal) an hour before you practice. Be sure you get your physician's approval before doing this. After some successful sessions have boosted your confidence, see how well you work without the medicine. If the problem is still just as bad, even when you have overcome your anxiety, it could be that microsurgery is not for you.

Do not, under any circumstances, use a tranquilizing agent to overcome a tremor problem.

HANDLING THE NEEDLE WITH THE NEEDLE-HOLDER

Put the straight jeweler's forceps (No.3) in your left hand and the needle-holder in your right hand. Use a 100-micron, flat-bodied microvascular needle with not more than 12 cm of thread (10/0 nylon) attached. When you are not suturing, park the needle on the sticky side of a piece of adhesive tape, doubled over. When picking up the needle from the sticky patch, get hold of the needle—do not pull on the thread.

GETTING HOLD OF THE NEEDLE WITH THE FORCEPS

At first grasping the needle is difficult because it is highly unstable in the needle holder and jumps around so that it points in any direction other than the one you want. The best way to pick up the needle is to proceed as follows.

Get hold of the thread with the left-hand forceps at a point 2 to 3 cm away from the needle (Figure 3-3, *A*).

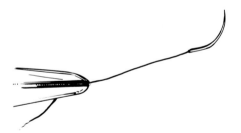

Fig. 3-3, A

Dangle the needle until it just comes to rest on the surface below (Fig. 3-3, *B*). It can now be made to swing around to point in any direction, and the angulated (right-hand) forceps can easily get it (Fig. 3-3, *C*). This can be done with the naked eye on a

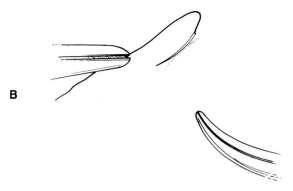

B

Fig. 3-3, B

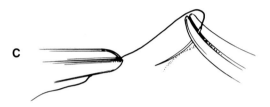

C

Fig. 3-3, C

white surface, or under the microscope. If the needle is still not pointing in quite the right direction, you can make minor corrections either by touching the needle with your left-hand forceps or else by partially relaxing your grip and nudging the needle tip against another firm object. You will soon learn that your needle is in a *stable* poisition if is it set up at 90° to the axis of the tips of the forceps (Fig. 3-4, *A*). The needle is *unstable* if its long axis deviates much from this position (Fig. 3-4, *B* and *C*). If you are using a flat-bodied microvascular needle, the problem of needle stability is not as severe.

In addition to getting the needle to point in the right direction it is also important that you hold the needle at the right point along its length. If you hold it too near the tip (Fig. 3-5, *A*), it will point downward. If you hold it too near the thread end (Fig. 3-5, *C*), it will point upward. *The needle tip should point horizontally, not upward nor downward.* Therefore you should hold the needle just behind its midpoint (Fig. 3-5, *B*). An upward-pointing tip only produces

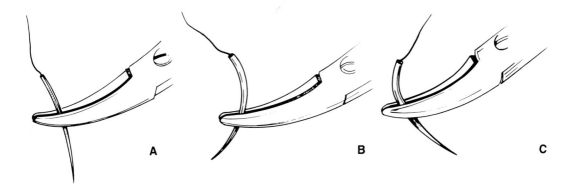

Fig. 3-4

inconvenience, but a downward-pointing tip produces a very real danger and you should strongly avoid it. When you do an anastomosis, there is serious risk that the downward-pointing needle tip will go through not only the wall of the vessel that you want to suture but also through the opposite wall. The result is a "through-stitch," which is one of the fundamental faults of anastomotic technique.

Sometimes to get the needle set up in the right-hand forceps correctly, you will have to pass it from one instrument to the other. Whenever you do this, let go with one instrument as soon as you have it with the other. If you hold onto the needle with both instruments at once, you will easily break it.

Whenever you start to pass the needle, get it set up

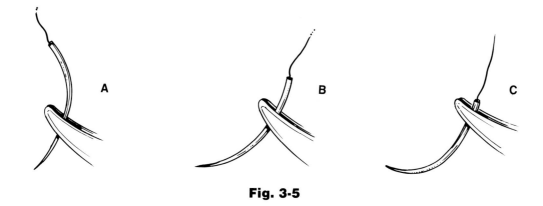

Fig. 3-5

in the needle-holder pointing right in the line it is intended to travel. Otherwise, you will find yourself trying to make a delicate and crucial adjustment just when things are getting difficult.

POSITION OF THE NEEDLE-HOLDER

The position in which you hold the needle-holder depends on the direction in which you are going to make your needle travel. In the natural "forehand" position, the needle-holding forceps is held with the tips pointing away from you and toward the left. This is suitable for passing the needle from top right to bottom left. You must not restrict yourself to this one position, or your style will be confined to working under artificially easy conditions. As your initial practice sessions progress, you must rotate the direction of your suture line around the clock in order to learn the various positions (See Fig. 3-17).

Changing direction is done partly by rotating the needle-holder around its long axis and partly also by altering the position of the hand. When the hand position is shifted, the main change is in flexion or extension of the wrist. The position of the fingers stays relatively unchanged.

Practice handling the needle in each rotation position of the needle-holder, and you will soon see that the needle can be made to point in just about any direction you want. Also, practice flipping the needle-holder quickly around from forehand to backhand. You will often have to do this when tying knots in order to pick up the thread easily.

PASSING THE NEEDLE THROUGH TISSUE

The needle should pass through the tissue perpendicular to the surface of the tissue. To achieve this, the tissue edge must be everted a little to provide the distortion that is necessary (Fig. 3-6). Eversion is produced by placing the tips of the left-hand forceps on the underside of the tissue and gently pushing the tissue edge up into eversion while spearing the tissue with the needle simultaneously.

Do not grab the thickness of the tissue between the

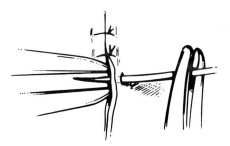

Fig. 3-6

jaws of your left-hand forceps in order to bring it into the position you want. This is a serious breach of atraumatic technique and should be avoided at all times, even on glove rubber. If you cannot bring the tissue edge up into eversion by the method recommended, two alternate methods are available. One is to pick up the next adjoining suture and lift it gently, which will often produce something approaching the desired effect. The other is to pick up not the thickness of the tissue but the surface of the tissue at a point a little distant from the actual tissue edge. This can be done with rubber, but it is a good deal easier to do with vessel wall tissue because there is always a little fibrous adventitia that you can pick up to produce the desired elevation of the vessel edge.

The needle must also come out the other side as nearly perpendicular as possible. Put the tip of your left-hand forceps on the top side of the tissue just beyond the place where the needle is going to come through (Fig. 3-7). Then when the needle

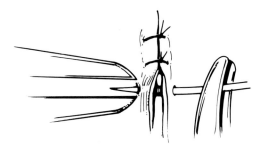

Fig. 3-7

comes through, it will bend the tissue upward as it comes out and pass through it perpendicularly.

The width of the "bite"—the distance between tissue edge and the needle hole—should be about three times the thickness of the needle itself. The bite on one side should be equal in width to the bite on the other side, and your needle should cross the suture line not diagonally but exactly at right angles (Fig. 3-8).

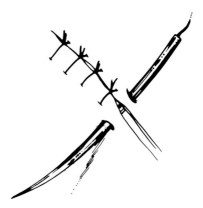

Fig. 3-8

Do not feel at the outset that you have to put the needle in one side and bring it out the other side all in one movement. This will come after a little practice. Rather, pass the needle through the first side and bring it out completely; then pass it through the second side as a separate maneuver.

When bringing the length of the curved needle through the tissues, *let it follow its own curvature* (Fig. 3-9, *A*). Pull it through with two or three short, straight pulls. Do not attempt to pull it through in one straight movement because this can cause gross distortion of tissue and unnecessary enlargement of the needle hole (Fig. 3-9, *B*).

CHANGING MAGNIFICATION

When you have passed the needle through both sides using high magnification, hold the needle in your left-hand forceps and pull the thread through.

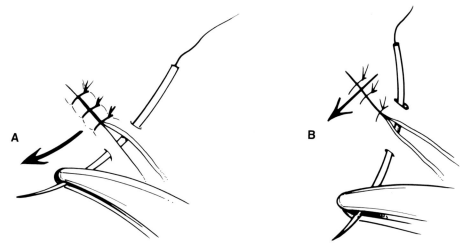

A

B

Fig. 3-9

Change to low magnification at this point so that you can see the end of the thread coming.

PULLING THE THREAD THROUGH

Keep the thread parallel to the direction of the entry-exit line as it comes through, using the tip of the right-hand forceps as a guiding pulley (Fig. 3-10, A). This avoids damage to the tissue caused by

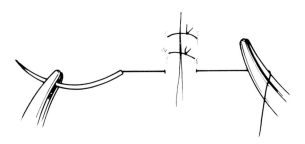

Fig. 3-10, A

angulation of the thread at the entry hole (Fig. 3-10, B). When the end of the thread comes into view,

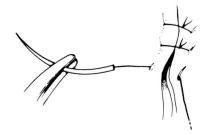

Fig. 3-10, B

stop pulling and let the needle drop. It is not necessary to see where it falls. The short end of the thread should be about 3 mm long. Get any redundant coils of thread completely out of your field of vision before you start tying the knot.

TYING KNOTS

Learning to tie knots in fine nylon is one of the principal sources of frustration in learning microsurgery. When you see it being done by an expert, the movements are fluent, rapid, and effective. Yet when you first try it yourself you will encounter every kind of entanglement and exasperation.

Tying a knot consists of four separate actions, and each of these presents its own particular difficulties. First, the thread is picked up with the left-hand forceps; second, a loop is made on the tip of the right-hand forceps; third, the short end of the thread is picked up with the right-hand forceps; and fourth, the loop is pulled off the right-hand forceps and the knot is tightened.

PICKING UP THE THREAD WITH THE LEFT-HAND FORCEPS

If you passed the needle through the tissues from right to left, you now have on the right of the suture site a short end of thread and to the left of the suture site a much longer length of thread that disappears out of sight. Take hold of the longer length of thread with the tip of the left-hand forceps about 1 cm from the suture site. The length of thread that now lies between your left-hand forceps and the suture site will be referred to as the "loop length." The loop length should be three times as long as the short end.

When you pick up the thread with your left-hand forceps, *pick it up so that the part that you are going to tie with, the loop length, comes out from the side of the forceps which is toward you (Fig. 3-11, A).* This makes knot-tying ten times easier. If you have the loop length coming out from the side of the forceps that is away from you (Fig. 3-11, *B*), then it is difficult to make it into a loop on the right-hand

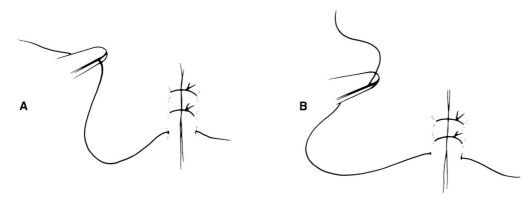

Fig. 3-11

forceps and, even when you succeed in doing this, the loop will constantly have an urge to fall off the forceps. If you start by picking up the thread with the left-hand forceps in the correct manner, these difficulties do not arise.

MAKING A LOOP   Having picked up the thread correctly in the left hand, it is usually simple to turn it in a single loop around the tip of the needle holder (Fig. 3-12). Sometimes this is done by winding the forceps

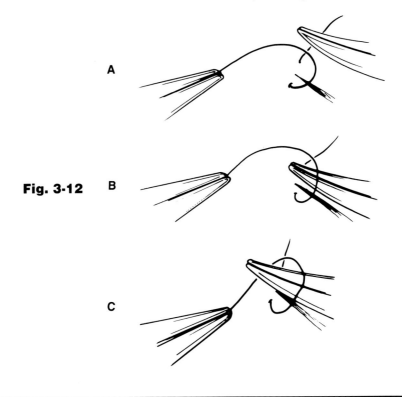

Fig. 3-12

around the thread, and sometimes it is achieved more easily if the thread is wound around the needle-holder. Most often a combination of these movements is used.

Put the loop well onto the tip of the needle-holder and keep it loose. If it is too near the very end of the needle holder or if it is too tight, it will easily fall off. Do the loop making quite near to where the short end is lying; then you will not have to carry your loop any distance before you pick up the short end.

A final pitfall in loop making is that when the loop has been made and the needle-holder holding the loop has been opened, ready to pick up the short end, the loop can fall off not both but just one of the jaws of the needle-holder, ending up between the two jaws. If you do not notice what has happened, and you go ahead and pick up the short end, you will find yourself in strenuous difficulties when you try to slip the loop off the right-hand forceps, because it will be caught between the jaws.

PICKING UP THE SHORT END

If the short end sticks up in the air cooperatively, there is never any difficulty in getting hold of it with the needle-holder (Fig. 3-13, *A* to *C*). More often than not, however, certain difficulties will present themselves: (1) the end may be too short, (2) it may be at an awkward angle, (3) it may be hidden, or (4) it may be lying on a flat surface. When you encounter one of the above, *do not* make repeated similar attempts to pick it up. Look at the situation. Analyze the difficulty and take action to alleviate it. Then go ahead and pick the end up— easily.

There are specific ways to correct or avoid the above difficulties.

If the short end is too short, pull it out longer. The usual reason for the end being too short is that you started out making the loop length too short and then

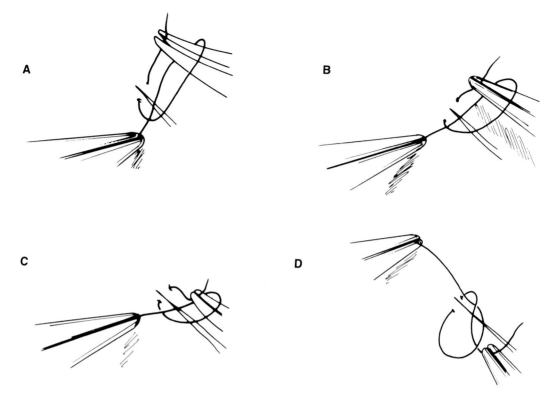

Fig. 3-13

pulled some of the short end through when making the loop.

If the thread is at an awkward angle for your needle-holder to pick it up, (Fig. 3-14, *A* and *B*) turn

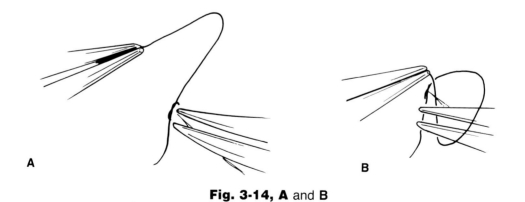

Fig. 3-14, A and B

the needle-holder around until it is at an angle where it will pick up the thread easily. It is a good deal simpler to make this change in the position of the needle-holder *before* rather than after you have made the loop. Therefore it pays to take a look at the short end and see how it is lying, before you start making your loop. Determine the best way to point your needle-holder so that you will be able to pick up the short end easily when the time comes. Put your needle-holder into this position, *then* make the loop and then immediately you can pick up the short end without difficulty (Fig. 3-14, *C* and *D*). If you do it in

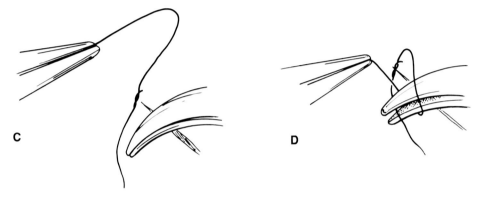

C   D

Fig. 13-14, C and D

this way, you will not have to accomplish an awkward change in the position of the needle-holder once you have made the loop.

If the short end is hidden or if it is obstinately stuck by surface tension to a flat surface, get hold of the short end with both pairs of forceps and bend it vigorously into a tight right-angle kink. This kink will stay and will provide you with a place where the thread can easily be picked up.

Often, when severe difficulties arise, it is wiser to drop your loop altogether and use both instruments to get the short end into a better position and then start the knot over again under friendlier circumstances.

Once you have picked up the short end, pull it gently through the loop with the needleholder (Fig. 3-13, *C* and *D*).

COMPLETING THE FIRST HALF KNOT

As you do so, allow the loop to fall off the tip of the needle-holder, and your first half-knot is made. Draw it to a gentle but not final degree of tightness.

Do not let go of the thread with the left hand. Hold on to it so you can go ahead and make the loop for the second half knot.

THE SECOND HALF KNOT

In making the second half knot, the sequence of movements—making the loop, picking up the short end, and pulling the short end through the loop—is repeated. Much of the exasperation of knot tying arises from trying to pick up the short end from a position of disadvantage (Fig. 3-14, *A* and *B*). This is an even greater problem with the second half knot than with the first. Do two important things before you make the loop: first, turn the needle-holder and point it in a direction that will make it easy to pick up the short end (Fig. 3-14, *C*). Second, put the jaws of the needle-holder *near* the short end so that once you have the loop made, you will not have to make a long journey with the needle-holder to pick up the short end. Don't make the loop until the needle-holder is correctly poised. When you make the loop, bring the loop to the needle-holder, not vice versa. Then you can go straight to picking up the short end without a struggle, without turning the needle-holder around, and without making a journey (Fig. 3-14, *D*). The first hundred times you pick up the short end you will have to think hard about this. After that it will start to become automatic and you will forget what it was that you ever found difficult.

Having picked up the short end, pull it through the loop and the second half knot is made. Tighten the completed double knot, bringing it—by eye, not by feel—to the degree of tightness that just brings the tissue edges into contact.

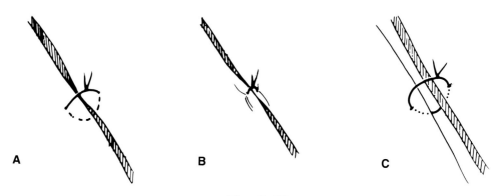

A   B   C

Fig. 3-15

The little circle of suture material enclosed within the tissue should remain visible (Fig. 3-15, *A*). If it disappears you have overtightened the knot and traumatized the tissue.

SLIDING THE KNOT TIGHT

If the tissue edges are a little unwilling to come together, tightening the second half of the knot requires particular care. Two things must be done: first, the tissue edges must be brought together, then the knot must be locked. If the knot locks prematurely, before the tissue edges are together (Fig. 3-15, *C*), the suture is useless.

There is a useful way of finally tightening the knot, which ensures that the tissue edges are brought together to just the right extent before the knot is finally locked. Start with both halves of the knot completely loose (Fig. 3-16, *A*). Pull steadily out to

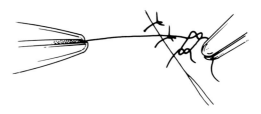

Fig. 3-16, A

one side on the short end only, keeping the long end slack (Fig. 3-16, *B*). The first half of the knot will

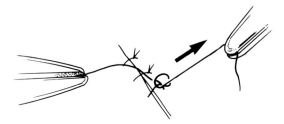

Fig. 3-16, B

progressively tighten, while the second half stays loose. Now, keeping up the pull on the short end, draw the other thread right across to the opposite side of the suture line and pull on it (Fig. 3-16, *C*); the second half of the knot will come tight.

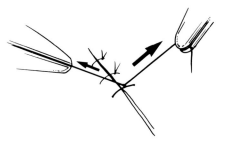

Fig. 3-16, C

HOW MANY HALF-KNOTS? Always use one extra half-knot for security, even when your first two have resulted in the best possible square knot.

If you used the sliding maneuver, your first two half-knots will give you "one straight thread and two half-hitches." For security this should be followed by two more half-knots.

RETRIEVING THE NEEDLE You can be sure of retrieving the needle, wherever you left it, if you cut the suture ends in the right order. Cut the short end first and discard it. Then hold onto the long thread and cut it close to the knot. Without letting go of the long thread, pull on it, and the needle will come into view.

The suture ends should be cut short and neat. If the ends are too long, they will get mixed up with the next suture. If you have made a neat square knot, your two thread ends will lie at right angles to the incision line and will not tend to stick down through the gaps into the lumen.

You should try to place two sutures per millimeter in initial practice exercises.

PROGRESSION OF EXERCISES FROM EASY TO DIFFICULT

To make things easy for yourself at the outset, you should first arrange the work so that the incision runs from top left to bottom right (Fig. 3-17, A). This

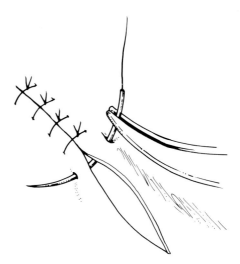

Fig. 3-17, A

enables you to hold your needle holder in the most comfortable and natural position. When you can suture easily in this position, turn the practice sheet around so that the incision crosses your field of vision horizontally (Fig. 3-17, B). In this position you have to both rotate your instrument counterclockwise in your hand and also flex your wrist a little to pass

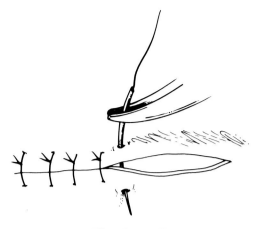

Fig. 3-17, B

the needle in the right direction. The next exercise, which is slightly more difficult, is to arrange the practice sheet so that your incision crosses your field of vision vertically (Fig. 3-17, *C*). Here you have to rotate the instrument clockwise and extend the wrist somewhat to get the right direction of movement.

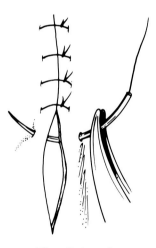

Fig. 3-17, C

Finally, when you find all these positions easy, go on to the most difficult of all, which is with the incision passing from top right to bottom left (Fig. 3-17, *D*). In this "backhand" position, it is best to hold the needle

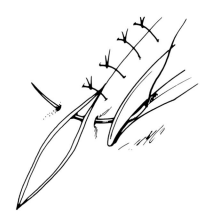

Fig. 3-17, D

holder with its points toward you, have the needle pointing backward, and suture away from yourself.

TOUCHING YOUR HANDS TOGETHER

When you are ready to attempt a more freehand working position, you must learn to work with your hands touching together. This is a useful way of diminishing unwanted movement when no hand support is available beyond the wrist. Touch the extended middle or ring fingers of each hand together with moderate pressure (Fig. 3-18). Then

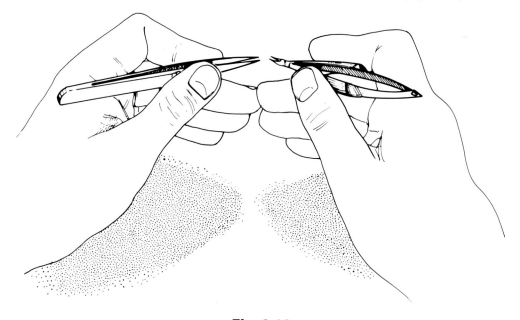

Fig. 3-18

rest your instrument-holding digits on the fingers that are touching.

To learn finger-touching you must be persistent. You may find that it feels unnatural and cramped at first. Most people do. Do not give up. After a few hours of mild discomfort, your hands will relax in their new relationship and you will have acquired an important extension of your skill.

TYING A SURGEON'S KNOT

In microsurgery, suturing under tension is often condemned, and rightly so. Still, there will be many times when you have to overcome the natural elastic retraction of tissues as you suture. For this, a surgeon's knot with a double throw on the first half knot is very useful. To cast a double loop give yourself an extra long loop length to work with. Place the double loop on the needleholder a long way from the tip to guard against its natural tendency to spring off the instrument. Once you can easily make a double loop you will find the surgeon's knot rather more secure and predictable in its action than the sliding maneuver shown in Fig. 3-16 (the only advantage of which is that the sliding maneuver lets you avoid double-looping when you are starting out).

SUTURING WITH YOUR LEFT HAND

There are rare but critical moments in microsurgery when your right hand has no way of passing the needle in the direction you want it to go. In preparation for such moments, do a little suturing with the roles of your hands reversed and learn to respect the competence of your left hand. It is not a stupid hand, in fact, with a little encouragement and praise you can get it to do almost anything.

chapter 4 Rat anesthesia and preparation

Rats are widely preferred for microvascular practice work. They have the advantages of being hardy, inexpensive, and easy to obtain. In addition they withstand prolonged anesthesia well. Rat vessels have thinner walls than human vessels and, in this respect, they are more difficult to work on. In addition, the femoral vessels are smaller than almost any vessels that will be encountered clinically. These factors will give you a certain theoretical margin of competence when you make the transition to working on human vessels. Conversely however, experience with the rat fails to simulate the difficulties of access, exposure, and control of unwanted movement that are often encountered in clinical work.

HANDLING OF RATS

Laboratory rats are clean and generally docile creatures. They become nervous and aggressive if kept alone in a cage and also if they hear loud, sudden noises. Rats dislike open spaces and are peaceful only if they are in close contact with things. They like to have their whiskers in contact with something.

Use rats weighing between 350 gm and 500 gm. Do not use a rat that makes wet, snuffly noises when it breathes or that has blood-stained nasal discharge. These are signs of mycoplasmal infection, and such rats are unfit for anesthesia.

Rat droppings can harbor worms that are transmissible to humans. Wash your hands if you touch them.

There are two ways to pick up a rat. You can take hold of its tail (do not hold it too near the end of the tail), or you can take hold of it behind the head with your index and middle fingers. Do this smoothly and firmly.

ANESTHESIA   The anesthetic agent used is pentobarbital (Nembutal) diluted in water to 6 mg per ml (one part standard injection to ten parts water). Shake the solution thoroughly. Draw 10 ml of the solution into a syringe and attach a 20-gauge needle with the beveled side of the needle downward and the graduated scale of the syringe upward. Discard any diluted Nembutal that is left over. It keeps poorly.

The cut-off sleeve of an operating room gown makes an excellent holding tunnel for the rat. Hang the sleeve over the corner of a sink so that the top end makes an inviting dark opening. Let the rat crawl into the sleeve. When its front legs have gone over the edge of the sink, get hold of the base of its tail and the scruff of its back through the cloth with your left hand and press its body (abdomen and legs protruding) into the corner of the sink (Fig. 4-1). Insert the intravenous needle obliquely through the center of the abdominal wall to a depth of 1 cm. Inject 1 ml of the pentobarbital solution per 100 gm of body weight. Put the animal back in its cage. It should be asleep in two to five minutes. Satisfactory anesthesia is indicated by quiet abdominal breathing,

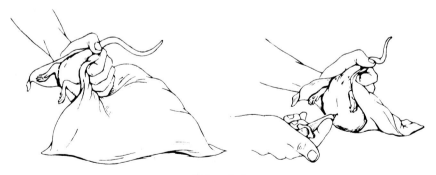

Fig. 4-1

a good pulse palpable on feeling the chest, and no response to painful stimuli.

Place the rat on its back and shave the upper part of each leg and inguinal region and also the entire center of the abdominal region, using the clippers.

Put the rat on the rat board. Wrap a piece of adhesive tape around each paw and put a push pin through the tape to fix the limb to the board. Have the limbs slightly outstretched (Fig. 4-2). Fix the tail to one side with tape. Attach a scalp vein needle to your anesthetic syringe, insert the needle into the abdomen, and tape it into position. Place a small blanket over the rat's body to prevent it from getting cold.

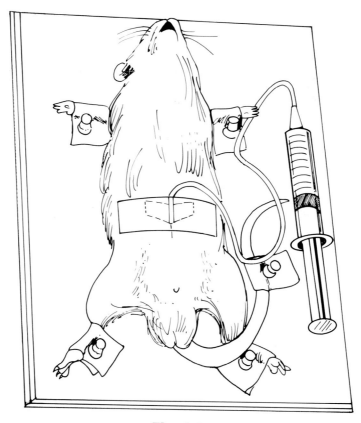

Fig. 4-2

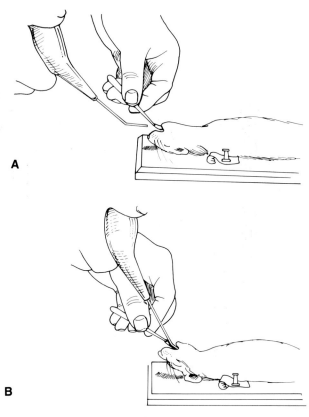

A

B

Fig. 4-3

If the rat develops respiratory distress during anesthesia, which is heralded by moist sounds from the airway and indrawing of the chest wall on inspiration, it needs to have its airway sucked out. To do this, get hold of the tip of its tongue with toothed forceps and pull the tongue out firmly (Fig. 4-3, A). Then take a dental chip syringe and, keeping the nozzle parallel with the neck, insert the tip of the syringe gently along the airway as far as it will go (Fig. 4-3, B). Suck out the airway while withdrawing and rotating the nozzle gently.

To sacrifice the animal at the end of an acute operation, inject 10 ml of anesthetic solution intraperitoneally or 2 ml intravenously. *Check carefully for complete cessation of pulse and respiration,* and check carefully to make sure you have not left any clamps in the wound before disposing of the animal.

chapter 5 Arterial anastomosis: common femoral artery

In this exercise, you will be learning to make an end-to-end anastomosis in a 1 mm artery. (When the diameter of the artery is mentioned, the dimension quoted is the external diameter measured with an eyepiece micrometer when the vessel is maximally vasodilated.)

As in many other jobs, the secret of success is preparation. The ease with which you can perform the anastomosis itself depends almost entirely on the care you have taken in each preparatory step. If you take trouble to give yourself good exposure, a bloodless field, and well-prepared vessel ends, you will have very little trouble doing the anastomosis itself. If, however, you hurry through the important preparatory stages and carry out each one incompletely, then your frustrations and difficulties will multiply until the job becomes impossible.

ANATOMY The common femoral artery is about 1.5 cm long. It starts at the inguinal ligament and ends at the point where it divides into superficial and deep branches. Just before its division, it gives off a large branch, the epigastric artery. The arteries are accompanied by corresponding single veins. Vein and artery lie within a common perivascular sheath.

SURFACE MARKINGS As you look at the leg, the vessel just visible beneath the skin is not the common but the superficial femoral artery. It emerges from under a layer of fat that lies beneath the skin of the inguinal area. This fat layer is an important feature in the exposure of the *common* femoral vessels: they lie beneath it. The epigastric vessels run laterally in the fat layer (which they supply). The inguinal ligament runs parallel to the concavity between the abdomen and the leg.

EXPOSURE   Make an oblique incision 3 cm long, through skin only, along the concavity between the abdomen and the leg (Fig. 5-1). Widen the resulting wound by pulling its sides gently apart with your fingers.

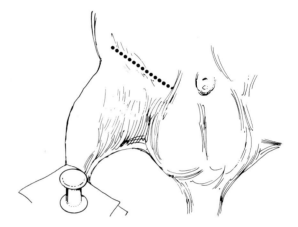

Fig. 5-1

You are now looking at the inguinal fat pad, and the next step is to reflect it laterally. Using microscissors and forceps, cut right through the fat layer around the upper, medial, and lower margins of the wound (Fig. 5-2, *A*). There will be bleeding from the branches of the epigastric artery in the fat layer as you do this.

Using the irrigating syringe and bipolar coagulator, locate each bleeding vessel, pick it up close to its divided end, and seal it. Aim for the vessel, not the blood, and be sure the grip of the forceps has arrested the bleeding before you apply the current. There is more about the bipolar coagulator further on in this chapter.

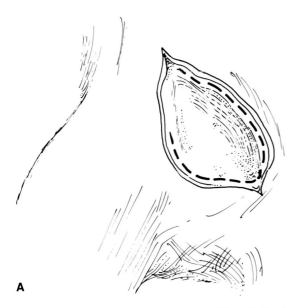

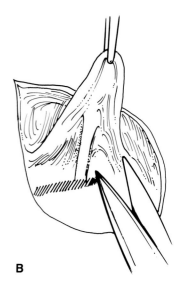

A

B

Fig. 5-2, A and B

Lift up the medial edge of the fat pad and pull it laterally (Fig. 5-2, *B*). It is bound to the underlying tissue by thin, filmy connective tissue. Incise this with microscissors, taking as much of it along with the fat pad as you can. As the fat pad is reflected laterally, the epigastric vessels are seen, curving up into it. They should be preserved. The common femoral vessels come clearly into view as you continue mobilizing the fat pad. Continue until you have the whole fat pad reflected and then leave it hanging over the edge of the wound (Fig. 5-2, *C*). It will be used later as a piece of soft tissue to press on the anastomosed vessel to produce hemostasis.

The common femoral vessels are now in full view within their perivascular sheath. The artery, of course, is the lateral one of the two. Lateral to the artery is the femoral nerve.

You are not yet looking at the whole length of the artery. Proximally there is more of it to be exposed, lying beneath the bulging muscle layer of the abdominal wall. This muscle is loosely bound to the

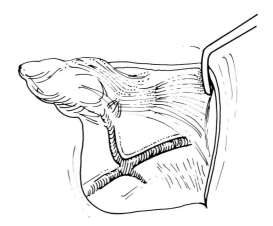

Fig. 5-2, C

tissues of the upper thigh by filmy adhesions, which must be broken down. Place a sponge over the femoral vessels and another sponge on the abdominal wall muscle. Put one thumb on each sponge and push the abdominal wall upward and medially until the white shiny inguinal ligament comes into view. Now put a wire hook retractor into the abdominal muscle, just above the vessels. Pull it with an elastic band over to the other side of the body and pin down the elastic band (Fig. 5-2, *C*). You now have the entire length of the common femoral vessels exposed.

Next, secure *complete* hemostasis right around the wound. *Do not go on until you have a completely bloodless field.*

VASCULAR DISSECTION

From now on, it is important to prevent the tissues from drying out. Moisten the wound every few minutes with Ringer's solution and mop away the excess with a sponge.

The next step is to incise the perivascular sheath over the artery and to free the artery from within it. First lift off and excise any remaining loose connective tissue that overlies the vessel. This loose tissue has many apparent "layers," but beneath it you come to a layer of tissue which is different in that

---

you cannot lift it up easily. This is the perivascular sheath. It envelops the artery and vein together, and the vasa vasorum run in it. There is a vague septum inside the sheath between artery and vein, and most of the vasa vasorum are here.

Take hold of the lateral part of the perivascular sheath with jeweler's forceps over the upper end of the artery (Fig. 5-3, *A*). Take the curved

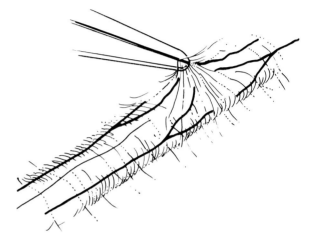

Fig. 5-3, A

microscissors and, holding them so that the blades lie *flat* over the artery, lift up the sheath and make a small hole in it (Fig. 5-3, *B*). Insert the underneath blade of the scissors in this hole and slide them along between sheath and artery, cutting as you go. Continue on down to the origin of the epigastric artery. At all times keep the scissors flat against the artery and parallel to it. If you don't, you run the risk of cutting the arterial wall (Fig 5-3, *C*). When incising the sheath, avoid cutting the vasa vasorum if you can. If at any time slight bleeding occurs, stop it with the bipolar coagulator and wash away all blood before continuing dissection.

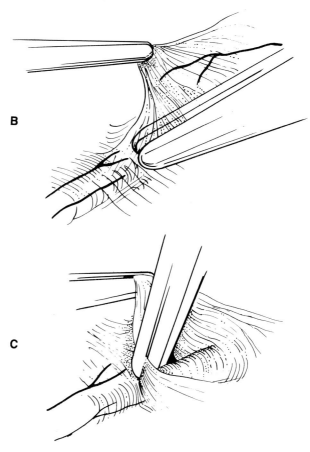

Fig. 5-3, B and C

Damage to the vessel during dissection will be avoided if you observe the following rules:

1. Do not work in a field obscured by blood.
2. Do not work out of focus.
3. Do not cut where you cannot see.
4. Do not hold the scissors at the wrong angle.

You are now about to touch the vessel for the first time, and here is an important point: *pick it up only by its outer layer, the adventitia* (Fig. 5-4). Never grab the whole thickness of the vessel wall. To be able to pick up the adventitia only, your forceps *must*

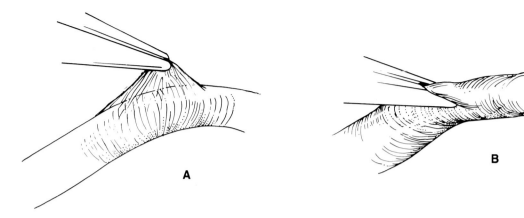

Fig. 5-4

be in good order. If they are not, take immediate steps to get a better pair, but first check to see that you do not have some small piece of tissue stuck between the jaws of the forceps preventing them from gripping exactly.

Now separate the artery from the surrounding vascular sheath. Pick up the artery with the jeweler's forceps in the left hand and gently divide the adhesions between it and the sheath. Use round-pointed scissors to do this, sometimes teasing and sometimes cutting. If you have a hard time cleanly separating the artery from its surroundings, almost certainly it is because you are not properly within the vascular sheath.

The lateral and medial side of the artery seldom give rise to any branches, but there is always one large, deep branch (sometimes more than one) that arises about midway along the common femoral and runs straight down into the muscle. Because its location follows Murphy's law of inconvenience, it has come to be known in our laboratory as Murphy's branch.

To divide Murphy's branch without a struggle, and without damage to the common femoral artery, first dissect 2 mm of it free. Pull the common femoral first to one side, then the other to give yourself a view of

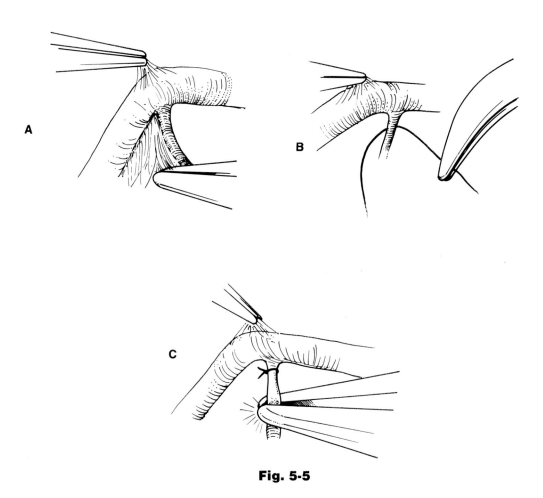

Fig. 5-5

what you are doing (Fig. 5-5, *A*). Then seal the branch distally over a short length (see below) and divide it with scissors (Fig. 5-5, *B* and *C*).

Now lift up the common femoral artery and dissect it completely free on the underside all the way from the inguinal ligament to the origin of the epigastric. Be thorough about this! If you don't have the vessel well-mobilized you will have major problems in applying the clamps and in turning the vessel over.

USE OF THE BIPOLAR COAGULATOR

The bipolar coagulator deserves a brief digression because it is one of the most important instruments in clinical microsurgery. The bipolar coagulator, unlike the regular "Bovie," has no ground plate. The current passes from one jaw of the bipolar forceps to the other. This minimizes the area of tissue subjected to heat damage. You can cauterize a vessel branch within a millimeter of the main vessel without any heat damage spreading to the main vessel itself. The bipolar must be used as a precision instrument. It works only if the vessel to be coagulated actually lies between the two jaws of the forceps. The main problem encountered with the bipolar is that the forceps stick to the tissue being cauterized. To avoid this, adjust the current to the lowest setting at which any visible cauterization occurs, always keep the tips clean, and avoid tightly grasping the vessel to be cauterized. All that is necessary is to gently surround it with the instrument tips.

Avoid bringing the bipolar forceps into direct contact with the main vessel when sealing a branch (Fig. 5-6, *A*).

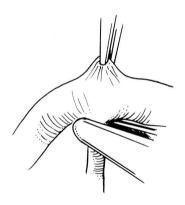

Fig. 5-6, A

You cannot rely on cauterizing one single point of the vessel before you divide it with scissors. Slide the forceps up and down the vessel so that a millimeter or two is uniformly coagulated (Fig. 5-6, *B*). While the bipolar forceps are being used on a branch, the main vessel should be held out of harm's way with a second pair of forceps.

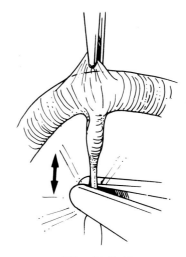

Fig. 5-6, B

Divide the sealed branch with scissors, placing the cut in the middle of the sealed length of vessel (Fig. 5-6, *C*).

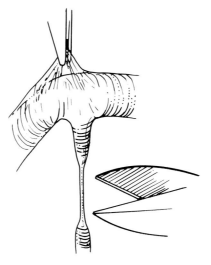

Fig. 5-6, C

SPASM   Your exposure of the artery is now complete, and the probability is that it has gone into spasm. Although "trauma" in general is blamed as the cause of spasm, the two main factors that seem to cause spasm are, firstly, cold, and secondly, contact of the outside of the vessel with freshly shed blood.

To relieve spasm apply 1% lidocaine (Xylocaine) to the vessel and wait three minutes. This interval is necessary because the time of action of lidocaine, although often less than this, is somewhat variable. Once good vasodilatation has been achieved, wash the lidocaine off with Ringer's solution (its continued presence in the wound promotes bleeding).

It is important that you do not proceed to the next step, clamping the artery, until the artery has regained its full diameter. If it is in spasm when you apply the clamps, then it will still be in spasm when you take them off on completion of the anastomosis. This is highly undesirable.

USE OF CONTRAST MATERIAL

Place a piece of blue plastic background material beneath the vessel. This makes the fine details of the vessel ends much easier to see. The vessel ends, once emptied of blood, are colorless and translucent. It is difficult to see them with precision and certainty unless a dark background material is used. Fig. 5-7 indicates the degree of improvement gained.

CLAMPING AND DIVIDING THE VESSEL

Move each clamp of the double clamp approximator to the end of its slide. Using the clamp-applying forceps, open one of the clamps widely and bring the approximator close to the artery. Lift up the artery and, sliding the suture-holding wire under it, bring the artery within the tips of the jaws and close the clamp. Open the second clamp and put the artery between its jaws. Just before closing the second clamp, pick up the artery between the clamps and pull up on it, bringing a little extra length of vessel to lie between the clamps.

With microscissors, cut transversely across the vessel midway between the clamps. If the origin of

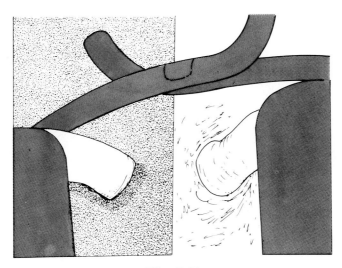

Fig. 5-7

Murphy's branch is anywhere near this point, excise the origin, together with a short length of the main vessel.

PREPARING THE VESSEL ENDS

You have three important things to do to each vessel end.

1. Get the blood out.
2. Remove the adventitia.
3. Dilate the vessel ends.

This preparatory work is extremely important. The care you take over it will, to a large extent, determine the quality of your anastomosis.

GETTING THE BLOOD OUT

It is not necessary to cannulate the vessel. Hold onto the end of the vessel with a pair of forceps and direct a fine jet of Ringer's solution from the irrigating syringe at the vessel end (Fig. 5-8). The blood in the vessel end will dissipate rapidly.

An alternate method of removing blood from the vessel end is to fold the vessel up and over onto the surface of the clamp and gently flatten it against this surface by milking with the tip of a pair of forceps. This should be done very gently.

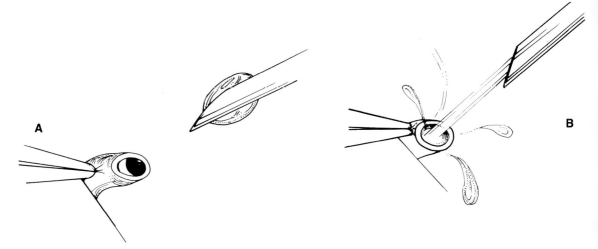

A

B

Fig. 5-8

There is no need to use heparin. There is no need to cannulate or medicate the artery in any way beyond the clamps. *Uncontaminated blood in undamaged vessels does not clot.*

REMOVING THE ADVENTITIA

Adventitia is the loose fluffy outer layer of white fibrous tissue. It is easiest to see when the vessel end is wet. It is important to remove adventitia thoroughly from the vessel end because, unless it is thoroughly removed, you cannot clearly see the cut edge of the layer that really matters for suturing purposes: the media. This is the only reason to remove adventitia.

Disregard the idea that you have to strip a whole length of vessel end. The idea is not to strip a great expanse of vessel but merely to trim the adventitia that actually hangs over the vessel end or that can readily be made to hang over it by pulling on it. Trimming the adventitia is best done with a pair of straight jeweler's forceps in the left hand and a pair of fine, straight, sharp-pointed scissors in the right hand. Take advantage of the fact that the adventitia lies loosely around the media like a shirt sleeve. Take hold of the adventitia with the forceps at the point on the vessel end closest to you. Pull this

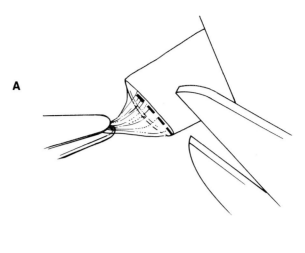

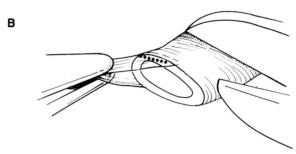

Fig. 5-9

adventitia off the end of the vessel by pulling gently in the long axis of the vessel. Keep holding on to it. The adventitia is almost transparent. Through it you can see where the end of the media is. Just by the end of the media cut through the adventitia with scissors (Fig. 5-9, *A*). This makes a hole in the adventitia. Put one blade of the scissors through this hole and cut first above and then below the site of the original cut until you have gone all the way around the circumference of the vessel (Fig. 5-9, *B*). While doing this, you must occasionally pick up the adventitia at a new place with your left-hand forceps in order to exert continuing tension on the adventitia that you are cutting.

The ease, neatness, and success of your anastomosis is largely dictated by the thoroughness with which you remove the adventitia from the vessel ends, so be patient and self-critical about it.

DILATING THE VESSEL END

There are two good reasons for dilating the vessel end. First, it converts the vessel from a piece of "spaghetti" to a piece of "macaroni"—a tube with a clearly defined wall and lumen that you can see and handle with confidence. Second, by stretching the smooth muscle of the vessel wall, you paralyze it for the next few hours. This effectively prevents spasm at the anastomotic site postoperatively.

The vessel dilator must be inserted and used with care. With microforceps in one hand, pick up the vessel close to the end, holding it only by the remaining adventitia. With the other hand, hold the vessel dilator so that the tips are pointing straight at the vessel end (Fig. 5-10, A), and insert the closed

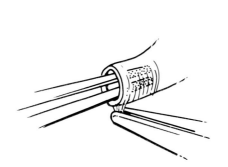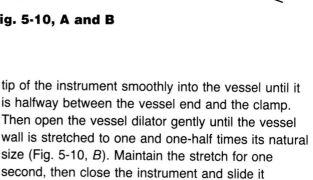

Fig. 5-10, A and B

tip of the instrument smoothly into the vessel until it is halfway between the vessel end and the clamp. Then open the vessel dilator gently until the vessel wall is stretched to one and one-half times its natural size (Fig. 5-10, B). Maintain the stretch for one second, then close the instrument and slide it smoothly out. See what a difference it makes in the appearance of the vessel end.

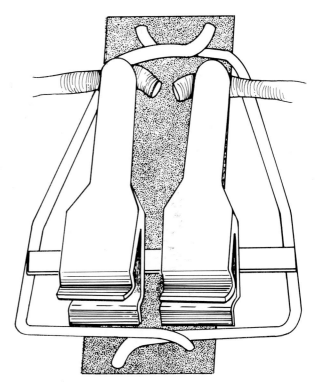

Fig. 5-11

Adjust the distance between the two clamps until there is about one vessel's width between the two vessel ends (Fig. 5-11).

SUTURING   The first two sutures, the stay sutures, are both the most important and the most difficult. They must be put, not opposite each other, but one third of the way around the circumference from each other. This ensures that when the stay sutures are pulled in opposite directions, the back wall of the vessel, being longer, will fall away, so that there will be no danger of picking it up while suturing the front.

Now, put in the first suture. Although for a time this suture will be pulled over to one side, you do not need to go right out to the "side" of the vessel to select the site for the first suture. Put it into the part of the vessel edge that you can see and handle most easily. Use the tip of your straight forceps for gentle counterpressure. *Do not grasp the thickness of the vessel wall with your forceps.* Remember to evert the vessel edge both at entry (Fig. 5-12, *A*) and exit (Fig. 5-12, *B*) of the needle so that the needle passes through the vessel wall perpendicularly. Concentrate on getting small, equal bites of tissue.

A   B

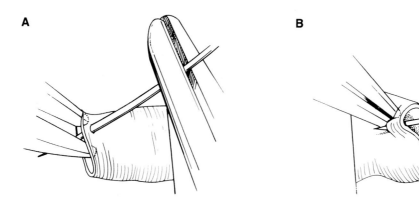

Fig. 5-12

Having made the entry bite, pause to see if you can make the exit bite easily without having to change your grip on the needle. If you need to make a change, drop the needle and pull its whole length through the tissue. Pick it up fresh in a better position once it is clear of the tissue, then go ahead and make the exit bite. When you become fluent in your technique, you will seldom need to make a suture in this plodding two-pass fashion, but in the early stages it is sometimes wise to do so. The alternative is to struggle to reposition the needle, while you have the entry side tissue delicately impaled on it. Such a struggle will always enlarge the needle hole and may even tear the needle right out of the tissue.

Tie the first half-knot with the very greatest care. If there is the slightest sign of excessive tension or unwillingness of the two ends to come together, stop tightening, bring the clamps a little closer together, and then continue tightening. If it looks as if there will be excessive tension and you persist in tying the knot tight, something will break—either the suture or the tissue. Make three consecutive half-knots. Leave one end of the thread long and wind it once in a figure-eight around the suture-holding "cleat" of the approximator frame which is *farthest* from you.

The cleat is best used in one particular way. Bring the thread over the middle of the cleat (Fig. 5-13, *A*), down, and around the lower of the two wire ends (Fig. 5-13, *B*). Then bring it horizontally across, up, and around the upper wire end. Having wound it around the cleat (Figs. 5-13, *C* and *D*), pull it gently to lock it into position, and cut the end off short.

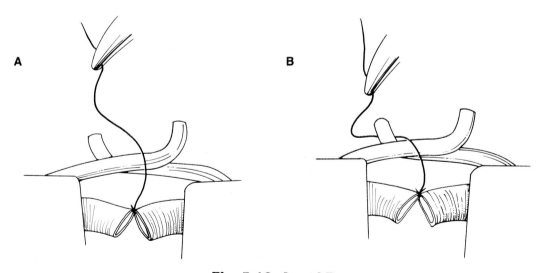

A   B

Fig. 5-13, A and B

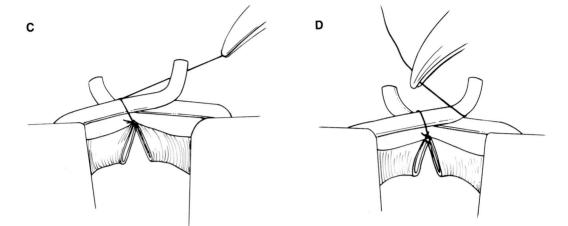

Fig. 5-13, C and D

The second suture needs the most care of all (Fig. 5-14). Carefully choose a point one third of the way around the circumference from the site of the first suture. Put the needle in, and with the greatest care bring it out the other side at such a point that both the entry and the exit points lie at equal distances from the site of the first suture.

If you successfully take one third of the circumference of one vessel end and match this with one third of the circumference of the other end, you will have made the start of an excellent anastomosis in which the edges will be evenly brought together all the way around the circumference. If, by contrast, you take one quarter of the circumference of one end and mismatch it with one half of the circumference of the other end, your anastomosis is destined to be crude, distorted, and unsuccessful. Therefore, the exactness with which you place *the second half of the second suture* is vital in determining the quality of your anastomosis.

Tie the knot, keep one end long, and wind it around the opposite cleat of the approximator. Pull on the thread gently, watching the anastomosis. When the tension on the second stay suture is such that the

A

B

C

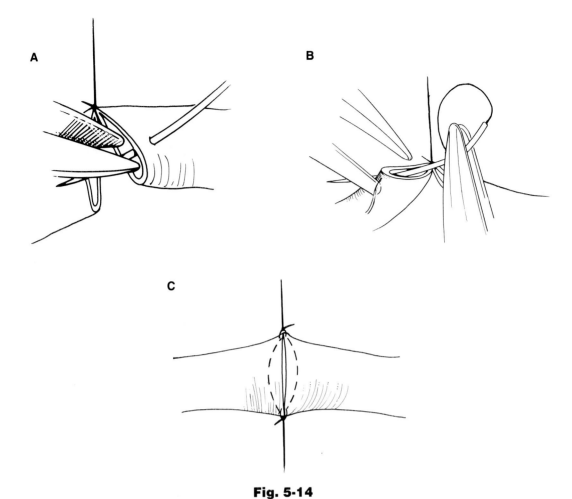

Fig. 5-14

two "front" edges of the vessel straighten out, lock the thread into the cleat.

By placing the two stay sutures in front of the "equator" of the vessel, you have produced a pair of short, tight front edges and long, slack back edges. The back edges will hang down out of the way of the needle as you suture the front edges. For the best effect, and the greatest safety, the back edges should hang not only down but also *back* from the anastomotic line. This is easily arranged by putting a little longitudinal tension on the anastomosis by suitable separation of the clamps (Fig. 5-15, *A*). If there is no longitudinal tension at all on the repair, the back edges will hang close together (Fig. 5-15,

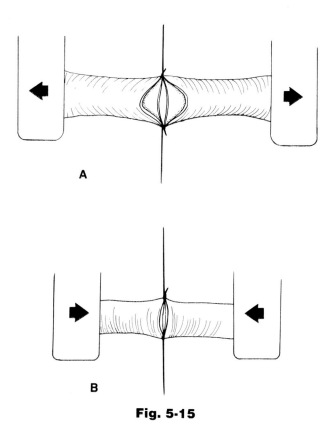

A

B

Fig. 5-15

B), and there will still be a danger of making a through-stitch which unintentionally picks up the back wall.

The front of the anastomosis is now set up so that it is very easy to suture. Put in two or three evenly spaced sutures to complete the front of the anastomosis.

As you progress toward completion of the row of sutures, the gap between the vessel edges becomes narrower each time you tie a suture, making each successive suture a little harder to put in. The last suture in the row is hardest of all because the edges lie so close that they cannot be separated. To avoid this difficulty, *do not tie the last-but-one suture,* but leave its ends loose while you put in the very last suture (Fig. 5-16).

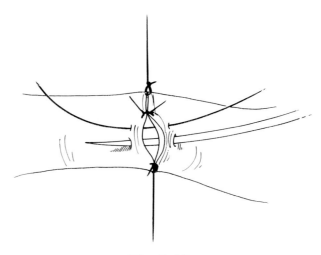

Fig. 5-16

Then tie both sutures. In this way the last suture is put in with a clear view of the lumen, and the danger of putting it in "blind" is avoided.

Now turn the whole approximator over. The stay sutures go over with it automatically. You are now looking at the long back edges, and you can see that they have stayed well out of the way of your front sutures.

Place the first suture on the back edges exactly midway between the two existing stay sutures. This is the useful *third stay suture* (Fig. 5-17, *A*). It divides

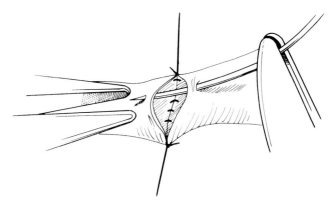

Fig. 5-17, A

B

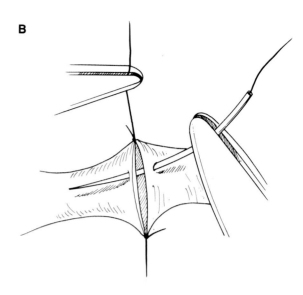

C

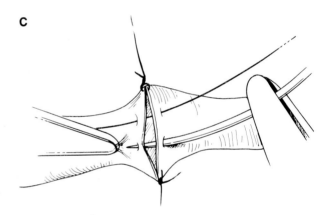

Fig. 5-17, B and C

the remaining unsutured part of the vesssel's circumference into two equal halves. Tie this suture and keep one end long. Attach the long end to the more distant of the two cleats. (It is not necessary to detach the one suture already held there.) Complete the suturing of the vessel edges that have thus been put on the stretch (Fig. 5-17, *B* and *C*), using two or three sutures, and again using the "untied suture" maneuver.

Now detach the third stay suture from the farther

cleat, bring it across, and attach it to the nearer cleat. The last third of the vessel's circumference is now ready to be sutured in just the same way as the first two thirds. When this is done, the anastomosis is finished.

AVOIDING A THROUGH-STITCH

A common cause of a blocked anastomosis among beginners in microsurgical technique is a through-stitch in which the far side of the vessel is accidentally picked up by the needle and included in the suture. On the front of the vessel this danger, though always present, is minimized by the proper use and positioning of stay sutures. On the back, however, you do not have this safeguard, and the danger of through-stitching is much greater. There are three important precautions against through-stitching. Observe all three, with every suture you put in:

1. Have the tip of your needle pointing horizontally along the surface of the vessel, never pointing down into it.
2. See where the tip of your needle is going—never guess.
3. Lift up the wall you are suturing, to separate it from the wall you are avoiding.

There are three ways of lifting up the wall. Either use the tips of your left-hand forceps inside the vessel to raise the wall, or pick up the adjoining suture and lift it, (Fig. 5-17, *B*), or pick up the adjoining adventitia and lift that (Fig. 5-17, *C*).

RELEASING THE CLAMPS

Having completed the sutures on the back side, turn the approximator back over, cut the stay sutures short, and unwind them from the cleats. Before you release the clamps, apply fresh lidocaine to the operative field, wait 3 minutes, then rinse it off. Remove the contrast strip from under the vessel. Release the rat's foot and reposition it so that the leg is flexed. This takes most of the natural tension off the vessel and helps close up the gaps and minimize leakage.

Release the clamps, first the distal and then the proximal one. Brisk bleeding will invariably follow. Do not be disturbed by this. As soon as you have the clamps off, bring the fat pad from the edge of the wound and place it over the vessel. Put a sponge on top of that and press gently but continuously for 2 minutes.

(NOTE: Rat vessels have thinner walls than human vessels of the same diameter, and for this reason they bleed much more.)

After applying gentle pressure for 2 minutes, quietly raise the fat pad and take a look at the vessel.

You are naturally anxious to know if your anastomosis is patent or not. *Do not* do anything to the vessel in the early minutes of flow in an attempt to assess patency. Just leave the vessel alone. It is difficult to assess patency in the first few minutes, and any manipulation of the vessel that you do at this stage can only serve to slow the flow and increase the possibility of thrombosis. It is during the early minutes of flow that the danger of thrombosis is maximal.

SIGNS OF PATENCY

To decide whether an artery is patent, first look at it and see how it pulsates. By intelligent observation you can often assess patency without handling the vessel at all.

One important point: pulsation proximal to the anastomosis does *not* tell you that your anastomosis is patent. You must look for pulsation *distal* to the anastomosis.

An artery can pulsate in three different ways: expansile pulsation, wriggling pulsation, and longitudinal pulsation.

Expansile pulsation. An increase and decrease in the diameter of the vessel is a sure sign of patency when seen distal to the anastomosis. Look carefully—expansile pulsation is not a very conspicuous movement, but it can be accentuated by a simple maneuver called the "uplift test," described below.

Wriggling. The alternating change in the curvature of a curved vessel that occurs with each pulse beat is called wriggling. (Wriggling is not apparent in straight vessels.) Wriggling distal to the anastomosis is a sign that the anastomosis is patent. Sometimes you can see wriggling in the curved epigastric artery even if it is not obvious in the parent vessel.

Longitudinal pulsation. Pulsation in the long axis of the vessel concentrated at a particular point means that the vessel is partially or completely blocked at that point. The column of blood in the vessel is "hammering" against an obstruction. If you see longitudinal pulsation at your anastomosis, it is a strong indication of partial or complete thrombosis. To confirm that it is blocked, apply the tests described below.

False wriggling. False wriggling consists of movement distal to a blocked anastomosis that looks deceptively like wriggling. This is a transmitted movement in the distal vessel set up by vigorous longitudinal pulsation at the site of the blocked anastomosis. To determine the true nature of the wriggling movement, hold the anastomosis still by taking hold of a suture. By stilling the longitudinal pulsation, false wriggling will be stopped.

TESTS OF PATENCY If you can see by observing these signs that the vessel is definitely patent, leave it alone. If you are in doubt, carry out the following tests, in the order given. *Carry out these tests distal to the anastomosis.*

Uplift test. At a point distal to the anastomosis, put a curved instrument under the vessel and gently raise it until the pressure of the instrument from underneath almost occludes the column of blood in the vessel (Fig. 5-18). Look closely at the vessel

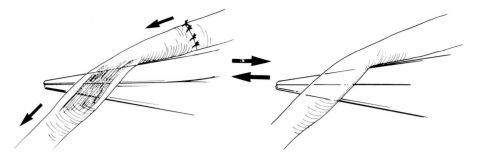

Fig. 5-18

where it crosses the instrument. If the vessel is patent, you can see it alternately filling and collapsing with each pulse beat.

Empty-and-refill test. This is a crude but definite test of patency that is traumatic and should be used as seldom as possible. With one pair of forceps, occlude the vessel distal to the anastomosis (Fig. 5-19, *A*). With a second pair of forceps, empty a

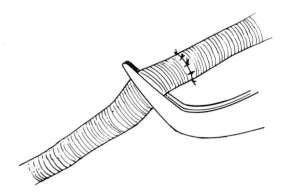

Fig. 5-19, A

short length of vessel distal to the first pair (Fig. 5-19, *B*). Then, holding the second pair of forceps closed, release the proximal pair and see if the emptied length of vessel refills (Fig. 5-19, *C*). Be sure that both pairs of forceps used for this test have parallel closing jaws. If they meet at an angle they

B

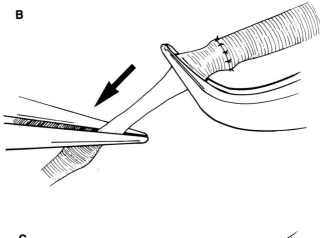

C

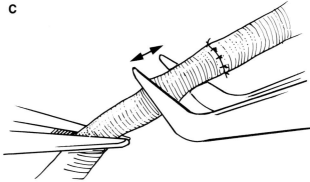

Fig. 5-19, B and C

will not produce convincing occlusion or emptying of the vessel. Be sure to do the empty-and-refill test distal to the anastomosis, and to do both the emptying and the refilling in the natural direction of flow. Otherwise the test will give rise to misleading information.

The ultimate test. Take a pair of scissors and divide the vessel distal to the anastomosis.

COMMON PITFALLS

1. Failure to get wide open access:
   − incision too small or wrongly placed
   − overlying fat pad not well mobilized
   − inguinal ligament adhesions not separated
   − retraction insufficient
2. Working in a blood-filled wound or on badly blood-stained tissues.
3. Dissecting out the vessel in the wrong plane.
4. Not mobilizing enough vessel.
5. Doing the anastomosis close to the unexcised stump of Murphy's branch.
6. Having the two clamps set too far apart (excessive tension) or too close together (poor view of lumen).
7. Not having vessel ends long enough to work on.
8. Incomplete trimming of adventitia leading to a poor view of the vessel edge and subsequent inaccuracy in suture placement.
9. Faulty placement of the second suture exit bite leading to bad coaptation all the way around.
10. Through stitching (see p. 71).
11. Imprecise suture placement.
12. Struggling to reposition the needle while it is on its way through the tissues.

chapter **6** Venous anastomosis: common femoral vein

Wait until you can anastomose arteries beautifully before you think about doing veins. Veins are harder than arteries—much harder. There are four reasons for this.

First, when dissecting out a vein it is harder to find the right plane between the perivascular sheath and the vessel wall. If you stray inside the plane you cut the vessel wall; if you get outside it, you end up with the dissected vessel swathed in loose tissue that is difficult to remove. The reason the dissection is so hard is because venous adventitia is different. With the artery, the easy plane of dissection lies anywhere within the thickness of the loose and abundant adventitial layer. Around the vein, the adventitia is neither loose nor abundant, so the plane of dissection is harder to find.

Second, the wall of the vein is easier to damage, whether by scissors approaching too close at the wrong angle, or by forceps, failing in the attempt to pick up the vessel by "just the adventitia." The wall of the vein is also disrupted with special ease at the site of any branch, if you are at all rough in pulling on the branch.

Third, the wall of the vein is thin, floppy, and easily distorted, making it hard to decide just where the edge lies and just where the needle tip should go.

Lastly at the site of any small insult or inaccuracy,

the amount of platelet thrombus that forms is greater in a vein that in an artery. Since flow is slower, platelets have more time to react to the site of injury and more time to stick to it.

DISSECTING OUT THE VESSEL

At the outset, check that your straight jewellers forceps meet precisely at the very tip. Start off on a previously unoperated side of the rat, not one where the artery has already been worked on.

From the very start, be more gentle. At the stage of initial access, when you have to separate the abdominal wall muscle from the tissues of the upper leg to expose the proximal vessel, refrain from using force. With the artery the instruction was to shove the abdominal wall upward. Not so when you're doing a vein! There is a branch vein in the abdominal wall that can be damaged by that rough maneuver, leading to occlusion of the main vein. So to displace the abdominal wall, retract it upward and medially, dividing all filmy adhesions not with force but with scissors until the inguinal ligament comes into view.

Next identify the vascular sheath and get inside it. Remember that the vasa vasorum run within the sheath. Clear away any areolar tissue that has no connection with the vasa vasorum. The sheath is the layer that, when picked up, brings the vasa vasorum up with it (Fig. 6-1, A). Get hold of the sheath, tent it up over the vein, and make a hole in it with the tip of the dissecting scissors. Have the scissor blades flat against the vessel as you do so. Let go of the sheath where you first held it and pick up the edge of the hole you have just made (Fig. 6-1, B). Put the underneath scissor tip inside the hole (Fig. 6-1, C). Using the scissor tip of a probe, define and open a space between the sheath and the vessel. Now develop this space along the length of the vessel, dividing the sheath as you go along.

Alternately probe and cut. Probe to clear the sheath from the vessel, then cut the sheath that you just

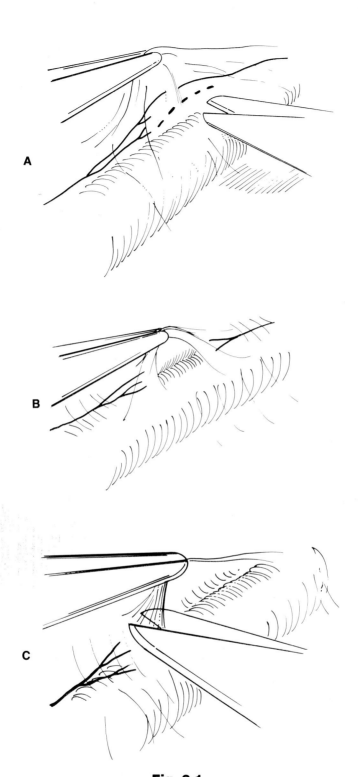

A

B

C

Fig. 6-1

cleared. Each time divide a little less sheath than you cleared with your probing. This will prevent you from accidentally cutting the tented up vessel wall.

Divide the sheath all the way from the inguinal ligament to the origin of the epigastric. Next free the vein from the sheath on the near side, on the far side, and finally on the underside. To free the near and far sides, pick up the near edge or the far edge of the divided vascular sheath and push the vein away from the sheath with the closed scissor tips (Fig. 6-2). On the far side, the sheath of the vein consists of the septum of loose tissue that lies between artery and vein.

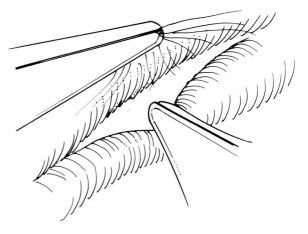

Fig. 6-2

Until now your handling of the vessel has amounted to nothing more than gently pushing on it with your rounded scissor tips. Now, to free it on the underside, you have to pick the vein up for the first time. The golden rule "handle the vessel only by the adventitia" applies with special force to veins, but there is so little adventitia to pick up that you may find the rule hard to follow. To get a good grip of that scanty layer of adventitia, proceed as follows. Apply the tips of the forceps, slightly open, to the surface of the adventitia (Fig. 6-3, *A*) and scoot them along the

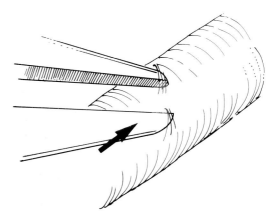

Fig. 6-3, A

vessel a short way so that a little wad of adventitia gathers up between the tips. Bring them together and you will have something worth holding onto (Fig. 6-3, *B*). With this you can readily lift the vein and free it from its surroundings on the underside (Fig. 6-3, *C*).

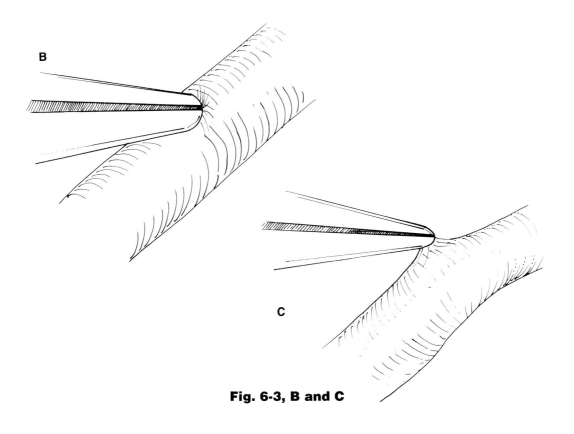

Fig. 6-3, B and C

Leave the branches that enter the vein on the underside until you have the rest of the mobilization completed. Free these branches from their surroundings with great patience and the least possible force. If you have an urge to stick your scissor tips into a blind spot here and there and let them fly open, resist it. That is a sure way to tear some small unseen branch. Instead staying always in the one good dissection plane, push the surrounding loose fibers away from the branch on all sides, cutting the occasional obstinate fiber. Pull as little as possible on the branch where it leaves the main vessel; it's a vulnerable spot. Ligate major branches with 10-0 nylon, flush with the main vessel. When using the bipolar forceps on tiny branches, turn the current almost to the lowest setting and keep the tips a millimeter from the main vessel.

Once you have freed the vein up completely, leave it alone with blood running along it for 10 minutes, then check to see if it contains any thrombi as a result of your dissection. To check this, place the tips of the angulated jeweller's forceps beneath the vessel distally, as in doing the "uplift" test, and slide them all the way along while closely observing the vessel at the point where the instrument occludes it. A thrombus is readily seen as a pale blob that stays in one place as the instrument slides by. If there are no thrombi, you did an excellent job of atraumatic dissection and you are ready to proceed. If thrombi are present, leave the vessel alone and take a 20-minute break. If they have dispersed by the time you return, proceed. If they are still there, abandon the vessel as unusable and start over with a fresh vessel, working even more gently than before.

Apply the clamps in the same way as for the artery. Don't hesitate to excise the stump of Murphy's branch if it will be in your way.

When you divide the vein, the two ends will look like sad pieces of stranded pond weed. Don't be discouraged. Even though they have no apparent form or lumen you will soon have them looking more hopeful. First, rinse the blood out of the lumen and remove all blood from every part of the wound by irrigation and suction. Then flood the wound completely with Ringer's solution. As soon as they are submerged the vessel ends will spring to a more life-like form. *Keep the wound flooded from now until the first two sutures are in.*

Next, bring in the piece of dark contrast material. Slide it temporarily into the space between the suture-holding frame and the clamps so that it is as close under the vessel ends as possible. Lastly, dilate each vessel end. Pick up the vessel edge by whatever adventitia you can find (Fig. 6-4, *A*) and poke around with one tip of the dilator until you locate the lumen. Insert the dilator, and produce a three-way stretch as shown in Fig. 6-4, *B* and *C*.

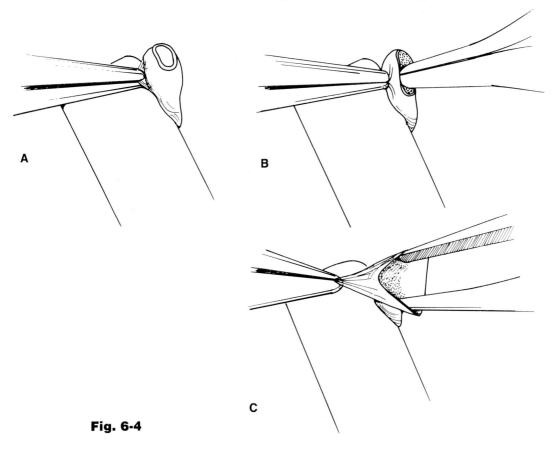

A

B

C

Fig. 6-4

Once you have stretched it, the vessel end will lose all its wrinkles and will look once again like a tidy piece of tubing.

If you dissected the vein out in the right plane, there will be almost no adventitia worth excising. What little there is will stay where it is, unlike arterial adventitia, which tends to wander. Only trim off pieces of loose material that clearly have an urge to intrude on the lumen.

As you get ready to put in sutures, keep in mind that it only takes one slightly inaccurate suture to produce failure. Most faults in suturing come from not seeing the vessel edge accurately at the moment of passing the needle. Be most particular about being able to see it with certainty each time you put the needle point in and each time you bring it out. To see the vessel edge with certainty, you need well-prepared vessel ends, high magnification, and a well-flooded wound. (If reflected light from the surface of the flood is disturbing you, change the angle of the microscope a little.)

The sequence of suture placement is just the same with the vein as with the artery. The right size of bite is indicated in Fig. 6-5, *A*. If you take a larger bite, tissue will get bunched up and distorted.

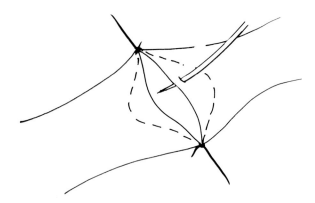

Fig. 6-5, A

B

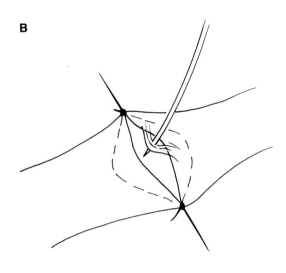

C

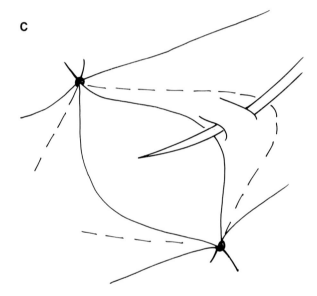

Fig. 6-5, B and C

The vessel edge has a tendency to roll inward. Because of this, two different errors are possible. With slight in-rolling, the needle tip can spear just adventitia (Fig. 6-5, *B*). With more in-rolling, the needle can go right through the vessel wall twice (Fig. 6-5, *C*). In either case the result is the same: raw, thrombogenic vessel edge hanging in the lumen.

To guard against unsuspected in-rolling, take the following precautions.

As you go to make the entry bite, pass the tip of the left-hand forceps well into the open lumen and bring it up under the vessel edge just beyond the point to be sutured. The moment you pass the needle, unroll the vessel edge gently, stroking it on the underside with a backward movement of the forceps (Fig. 6-6, A and B). Convince yourself that what you are looking at is a single thickness of vessel edge, then pass the needle.

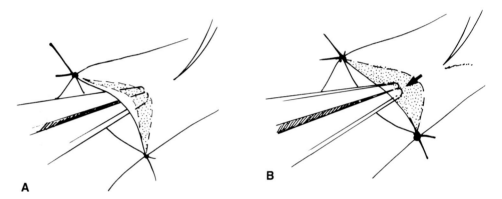

A   B

Fig. 6-6

Coming out, use the needle tip to do the unrolling. Pass it into the open lumen a little beyond the intended point of exit. Bring it up against the vessel edge and stroke the tissue with a backward movement to reveal and undo any in-rolling (Fig. 6-6, C and D). As you do this, have the tips of the left-hand forceps poised against the wall on the outside to provide counterpressure.

Put in the first two sutures *under Ringer's solution*. When you have the two stay sutures pulled out in opposite directions, the whole thing begins to be recognizable, and the rest of the anastomosis will be straightforward.

C

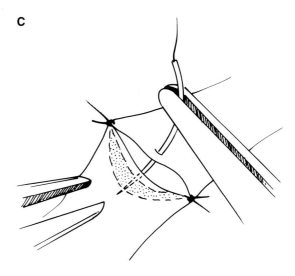

D

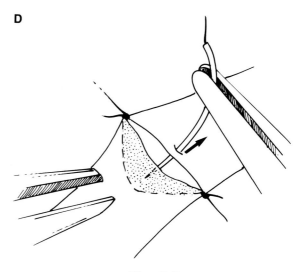

Fig. 6-6

The sutures in the vein can be twice as far apart as in arteries, because the pressure is so much less. As the vein is twice the diameter of the artery, you still end up with about ten sutures.

On completion of the anastomosis, omit the use of any vasodilator. Instead, be sure that you remove the distal (i.e., high pressure) clamp first, to blow the anastomosis wide open as flow begins. When you take off the clamps, the vessel should dilate fully at the site of the anastomosis. If the vessel remains constricted at the site of anastomosis, it is almost certain that at least one of the sutures of your anastomosis is a through-stitch. If this happens, reclamp the vessel immediately and wash the blood out from inside it by vigorous external irrigation and by "milking." Then find the offending suture, remove it, and replace it.

SIGNS OF PATENCY   If the site of anastomosis is well dilated and the vein proximal to the anastomosis is the same diameter and the same color as the vein distal to it, you can be reasonably certain that the anastomosis is patent. To check patency, use a gentle modification of the uplift test. Place a curved forceps beneath the vein just distal to the anastomosis, lift it up so the vessel is just occluded, and move it along under the vessel in a proximal (i.e., downstream) direction, going past the anastomosis (Fig. 6-7). If the vessel fills up

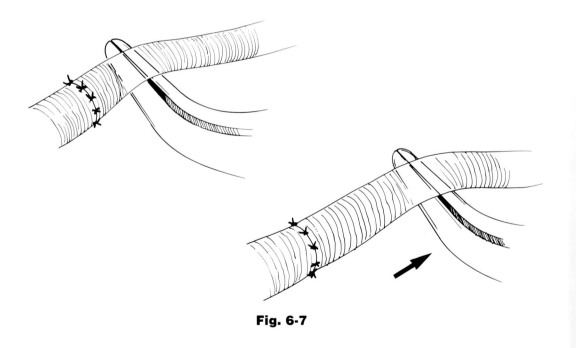

Fig. 6-7

briskly behind the moving instrument, then the anastomosis is patent.

If the vein is blocked, it will be more dilated distal to the anastomosis than proximal, the filling test will be negative, and in the course of time the blood in the vein will become extremely dark.

COMMON PITFALLS
1. Embarking on the vein before you are proficient on arteries.
2. Starting on a side which has already been used for the artery.
3. Dissecting the vein out in the wrong layer.
4. Damaging the vessel during dissection with forceps, with scissors, or with bipolar coagulator; or by pulling on branches.
5. Overhandling the tissue in vessel end preparation and in suturing.
6. Any minor fault in suture placement, especially if in-rolling of the vessel edge is produced.

chapter 7 Some practical points about blood—and some rules of practice

When blood inside a vessel is standing still, it will not clot unless the vessel is damaged or the blood is contaminated with thromboplastins. Uncontaminated blood in an undamaged vessel will remain liquid for several hours because the undamaged vessel lining secretes anticoagulant substances. When a cleanly dissected vessel is clamped and divided, the blood that is brought to a standstill above and below the clamps will remain liquid without any need for heparin.

If the vessel has been damaged, blood that stands still in it will clot. Such clotting will occur where a vessel has been clumsily dissected, where a branch has been cauterized too close to the main vessel, or where a clamp has been previously applied and then removed. These and other forms of trauma can all be avoided by the use of a careful, methodical, and precise surgical technique.

If the blood in the vessel has been contaminated with thromboplastins, it will clot rapidly, even in an undamaged vessel. Thromboplastins, which are soluble in water, are present in any fresh surgical wound. The irrigating fluid in a wound quickly becomes a thromboplastin solution. If it gets into a vessel that has blood standing still in it, clotting will occur. The practical point is that *blood that is in open contact with the wound should never be allowed to stand still in a vessel* unless the irrigating fluid contains heparin. In the laboratory heparin is not used in basic exercises, so take care to observe this important rule of practice.

Moving blood in a damaged vessel produces a platelet thrombus. The cause of early anastomotic failure is almost invariably platelet thrombosis and almost never whole blood coagulation. Whether a platelet thrombus occludes a vessel depends on the size of the thrombus relative to the vessel. A smooth and streamlined microvascular anastomosis that has been carried out with minimal tissue handling will produce a negligible quantity of thrombus in a 1-mm vessel. A crudely performed anastomosis full of gaps, irregularities, and overlaps will rapidly give rise to sufficient thrombus formation to occlude the vessel. The size of the thrombus depends not only on the severity of the damage (i.e., the crudity of the surgical procedure) but also on the rate of blood flow. A larger thrombus forms when blood flow is slow than when it is rapid.

Three main factors, therefore, determine anastomotic patency: the size of the vessel, the quality of the surgical procedure, and the rate of blood flow.

Clearly the ideal quantity of platelet thrombus to produce is none at all. Since we may sometimes fall short of this ideal, here are some points about small platelet thrombi that are worth knowing.

A small nonoccluding platelet thrombus is a transient object. A platelet thrombus, under conditions of continuous flow, has a distinct natural history, a rise and fall. It grows to a certain size, then stops growing, and then disintegrates. Its growth is complete within 5 minutes, it starts to disintegrate by 10 minutes, and by the end of an hour it has almost completely gone, leaving the site of injury covered with an inert coating.

This process depends on continuous blood flow past the thrombus. If blood flow stops before the life cycle of the thrombus is complete, then processes begin that cause the thrombus to become permanent. Blood flow will stop either because it is interrupted by surgical interference or because the thrombus has become large enough to occlude the whole vessel. The process which then commences and makes the platelet thrombus permanent is fibrin formation, that is, whole blood clotting in the space adjoining and surrounding the platelet thrombus.

Nonoccluding thrombi may be produced at two stages of a procedure. The first stage is when the vessel is dissected free of its surroundings. The second is the when the clamps are released on completion of the anastomosis. The risk in the latter period is the greater of the two. There are, therefore, two periods when it is wise to *leave the vessel alone and let it run:* for 20 minutes after the vessel is dissected, and for 20 minutes after the release of the clamps. If you stop the flow in a vessel that has a nonoccluding platelet thrombus in it, the thrombus not only will stop going through its natural self-disposing life cycle but also will give rise, during the period of stasis, to an attached whole blood fibrin clot that is much larger and that may well occlude the vessel.

A nonoccluding thrombus may be suspected when there is a slight longitudinal pulsation, or may be seen by lifting the vessel with a polished instrument and observing the appearance of the transilluminated blood column. Do not milk such a thrombus away by massaging the vessel. If it is going to disintegrate, it will do so only by being left alone. If you dislodge it forcibly and prematurely, a fresh thrombus will arise, and you will also have produced a sizable embolus that may go on to produce distant bad effects.

If, as you watch, a partially occluding thrombus grows and produces complete occlusion, only one course of action is likely to restore patency. Clamp the vessel, remove at least three sutures, instill heparinized Ringer's solution until the blood is all out, put the dark plastic behind the vessel to render it clearly visible, and take a long look to see what went wrong. Your action to rectify the situation depends on what you find and will range from the revision of a single bad suture to the complete excision of the anastomosed segment and replacement with a vein graft.

RULES OF PRACTICE
This seems a good point to bring together some basic and simple "rules of practice" for microvascular surgery.

1. Dissect the vessel cleanly with minimal handling.

2. Once it has been dissected, leave it running for 20 minutes.

3. Clamp the vessel and leave the clamp in the same place throughout the procedure.

4. Do not let blood stand still in an open vessel end or in an uncompleted vein graft, or in any situation in which blood in the vessel is in contact with a freshly made anastomosis or in communication with the wound. Either get rid of the blood or put heparin in with it.

5. Make a clean, smooth anastomosis.

6. Maximize vessel diameter by avoiding postoperative spasm.

   a. Minimize spillage of blood onto the outside of the vessel.

   b. Apply a topical vasodilator before applying the clamps and again before releasing them.

   c. Dilate the vessel ends physically.

7. Let the vessel run uninterruptedly once the clamps are released.

8. When doing an artery and vein together, complete both anastomoses before releasing any clamps, and then release all the clamps at the same time.

9. If after completion of the anastomosis the vessel has to be reclamped for any reason, wash out the blood standing in it so that it does not clot. (Do this by bombarding the suture line vigorously with a fine jet of Ringer's solution. It gets in through the gaps most effectively.)

chapter **8** Interpositional vein graft

Gaining the ability and willingness to do a vein graft when it is needed is an important step toward competence as a microsurgeon.

Wait until you have had repeated success with straightforward vein anastomoses before you try this exercise. The anastomoses of the vein graft are at least as hard to do, and many additional details demand attention.

The object is to remove a short length of the common femoral artery and replace it with a length of epigastric vein. Be sure you have a clear idea of the sequence of action before you start. In particular be clear about two matters which are described in detail later—the proper length of the graft, and the management of the clamps.

Start with a new and healthy rat. In addition to your double approximator clamp you must have two single clamps.

Give yourself a big, wide-open wound to work in. Make the regular inguinal incision, but make it a little longer than usual. Separate the fat pad, the abdominal wall, and the leg muscles from each other widely and thoroughly, not leaving any webs or bands of loose fascia. Take care not to harm the epigastric vein when raising the fat pad, because it is to be your graft.

DISSECTING OUT THE GRAFT

Dissect the vein graft free first so that it has time to sit and recover before you use it.

You may have been exposed to the idea that taking a vein graft is a piece of rough work to be delegated to a less-trained person and done under adverse conditions. This is a bad and dangerous idea: the damage that is done when it is carried into practice contributes to the general perception that vein grafts are a little chancy. In microvascular surgery, the need for dependable success dictates a quite different attitude toward the taking of a vein graft. It should be done as an exercise in fine microsurgical dissection, applying all the good habits of fine vessel handling that you have already learned.

You will be dissecting the epigastric vein out all the way from its emergence from the fat pad to its junction with the common femoral vein. To make this easy, first put the vein under a little tension so that it does not wander around while you deal with it. Engage a retractor in the fat pad, pull it out sideways, and fasten it down so that the vein is straight, but not narrow (Fig. 8-1).

Dissect off any overlying tissue and get down to the perivascular sheath. Over the vein pick up the sheath and divide it with dissecting scissors. Let go of it, pick up the edge of the window you just made, and put one blade of the scissors inside the sheath—parallel with the vessel and with the cutting edge away from the vessel wall. As you did with the common femoral vein, use the scissors alternately to probe and then cut, cutting always not quite as far as you probed so that you avoid puncturing the vessel.

If you cannot readily get into the plane of dissection, direct a vigorous fine jet of Ringer's solution at the window you made in the sheath. If the window does communicate with the plane of dissection, the Ringer's solution will get into the plane and open it wide for you all around the vessel and over a good length.

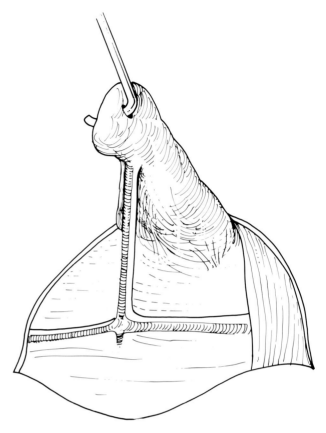

Fig. 8-1

With the sheath incised from end to end, methodically free the vein from its surroundings on the near side, the far side, and underneath. Use the bipolar coagulator, set very low, to seal any small branches. Once the vein is fully dissected, give it a good rinse and then restore it to its full diameter by raising the venous pressure. To do this, place a heavy thumb on the rat's abdomen and hold it there, occluding the vena cava until the pressure builds up enough to distend the epigastric vein.

PREPARING THE ARTERIAL DEFECT

Dissect the common femoral artery out of its sheath over its *entire* length. Proximally, free up the artery where it emerges beneath the inguinal ligament, retracting the ligament vigorously. Coagulate and divide the branch that arises just at this point. Distally, dissect until the origin of the epigastric artery is clearly seen.

Next, take two single clamps and place one as far up as possible and the other as far down as possible on the exposed artery. These are the upper and lower "guard" clamps. They will stay on until the very end of the procedure.

Now excise the middle third (not more) of the exposed artery, creating the arterial defect (Fig. 8-2, A). Empty the blood out of the divided ends and prepare them for anastomosis in the usual way.

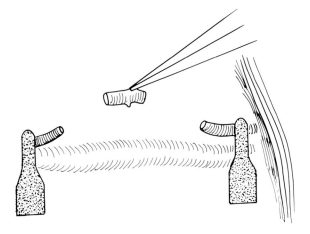

Fig. 8-2, A

CLAMPING AND CUTTING THE GRAFT

You are now going to take a measured piece of epigastric vein that is the same length as the arterial defect. Note that the length must be measured before, not after the vein has been divided (Fig. 8-2, B). When the vein is divided it immediately becomes much shorter. Its length will be abundantly restored as soon as it gets arterial pressure inside it. If you make the mistake of measuring off the "required length" on a piece of excised, collapsed vein, you will find at the end of the job that your vein graft is about twice as long as you wanted. This makes the graft tortuous, which is bad.

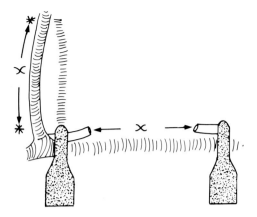

Fig. 8-2, B

Before taking the vein graft, think about one more thing. Once you divide it at each end, the graft will shrivel into a tiny, shapeless blob. This makes it extremely hard to handle, and putting it in a clamp can be a real struggle. To avoid this problem, it is a good idea to put a clamp on the vein graft *before* cutting it free, using for this purpose one half of the double approximator clamp that is to be used for the graft anastomosis. This clamp should go on the vein where it will be in just the right place to let you go ahead with your first anastomosis as soon as the graft is cut. With these thoughts in mind, you are ready to measure, clamp, and cut the graft.

To avoid a mess when the vein is divided, bipolar-coagulate the vein as high up and as low down as possible—but do not divide it yet. To measure the defect, take a pair of forceps and, using them like a compass divider, separate the tips so that they are the same distance apart as the two artery ends. Keeping the tips separated by just this amount, move them over to the vein and mark two points on the vein that will be the two ends of the graft. Mark each point with a small bipolar burn in the soft tissue adjacent to the vein. (If you trust your judgment well, you can do the measuring by eye.)

Take the approximator clamp and separate the two clamps quite widely. Open one clamp only, and apply it to the vein just two vessel widths away from one of the chosen end points of the graft. This end point should lie right between the two clamps. Note that to this time the vein has remained *intact*. Now, divide the vein (Fig. 8-3, *A*) at the two chosen points, and you have your graft (Fig. 8-3, *B*).

Empty the blood out of the short end of the graft by irrigation in the usual way. The long end is difficult to empty by irrigation. Instead, lay the graft on a soft surface and stroke it gently toward its open end with a smooth instrument.

Prepare the end of the graft that lies between the clamps for anastomosis by dilatation and minimal adventitial trimming. If your vein dissection was done well, there will be almost no trimming to do.

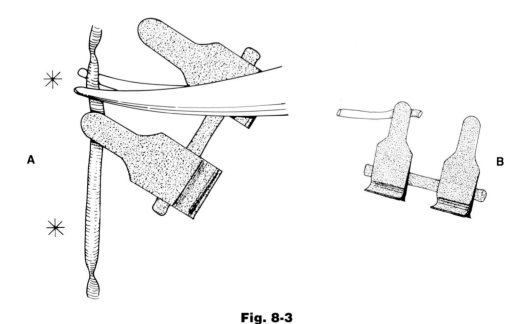

Fig. 8-3

FIRST ANASTOMOSIS   Now you are ready to do the first anastomosis. If you are right-handed, start with the one on the right. That way, each time you pass the needle there will be a little steadying contertraction provided by the attachment of the right-hand end of the artery to its surroundings. (If you did the left-hand anastomosis first, the vessel ends and the double clamp would run away from you each time you passed the needle because the double clamp would be drifting around freely in the wound).

I trust you can do straightforward end-to-end anastomosis quite easily now in arteries and veins. If so, you will find nothing unfamiliar in doing these anastomoses. You can use beginner's technique if you wish as in the preceeding chapters, or you may feel you are ready to move on a little using the slightly modified technique described here. This is a two-stay–stitch technique with turnover of the vessel but without the wire suture-holding frame and without the third stay suture.

For this you need to cut yourself a little "dumb assistant" out of background material shaped as shown in Fig. 8-4 and with two scissor cuts at each end to serve as suture holders.

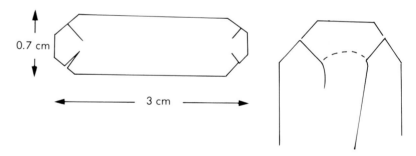

0.7 cm

3 cm

Fig. 8-4

As you prepare the vessels ends, dilating the end of the vein graft may present a problem because the two ends of the dilator may to be too big to get

inside the vessel both at once. If so, use just one at
first. Once you have got one end in and given a little
stretch, you can then get them both in and give a
real stretch. The secret of success in doing this is to
maintain a firm adventitial grasp of the vessel close
to the end with your left-hand forceps so that the
vessel end doesn't run away from you.

Put the stay sutures in at 120 degrees, keeping them
both equally long. Don't cut the "short" one
short—you will need it long when you turn the
vessel over. Fasten the stays to the dumb assistant,
using the scissor cuts as cleats (Fig. 8-5).

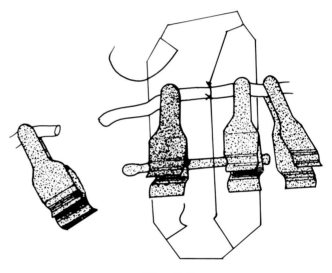

Fig. 8-5

With the near side sutured, unhitch the stays and
switch them over. On the back side, practice getting
along without a third stay suture. The vessel edges
are rather loose, but you can bring them under
control by tightening the tissue in one of two ways.
Either pull on the vessel edge, drawing it away from
the far stay suture to tighten it (this works well for the
first few sutures) or pull on the previous suture,
drawing it away from the near stay suture to tighten it
(this works well for the last few sutures).

SECOND ANASTOMOSIS   With the first anastomosis done, take off the double clamp but leave the single proximal guard clamp on (Fig. 8-6). You don't want to fill up the proximal half of your graft with blood at this point.

Before you put the double clamp on for the second anastomosis, make sure the graft is not twisted. Even a half turn of twisting in such a short graft will make it occlude. To check for twisting, take hold of the edge of the free end of the graft and gently pull on it. The vein will reveal any twist that it has by an uneasy rolling movement to one side or the other.

If you are using the double clamp with the suture-holding frame, take care, as you apply it for the final anastomosis, to ensure that you get the wire frame *beneath* both vessel ends. If you apply it beneath one end and above the other you will end up with the wire frame encircling the vessel in a quite perplexing way.

You can do the second anastomosis the same way as the first if you like (Fig. 8-7). Or if you are ready

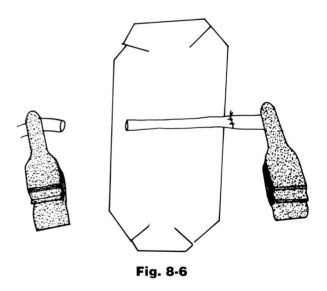

Fig. 8-6

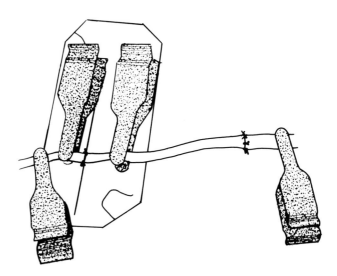

Fig. 8-7

for something more difficult, you can do it "one way up" as described in Chapter 9.

When both anastomoses are complete, remove the approximator clamp first; then remove both single clamps. Apply gentle firm pressure in the usual way.

COMMON PITFALLS

1. The graft can be the wrong diameter. We use the epigastric vein because, in its natural state, it is the same diameter as the femoral artery. A common mistake is to use too large a vein. This happens when we choose a vein which, *when collapsed,* looks the same size as the artery.

2. The graft can be the wrong length. The graft must be the same length as the gap in the artery—not longer or shorter. Measure it to this length while the vein is still intact, not after it is excised and collapsed.

3. The graft can get twisted. Remember to check for twisting before starting the second anastomosis.

4. Blood can get into the graft and clot while you are busy doing the anastomoses. Remember, the guard clamps stay on until *both* anastomoses are finished.

5. The graft can disappear up the sucker. This cannot happen if you put a clamp on the graft before excising it.

6. The cleat frame on the approximator can get locked around the vessel. You have a way out if this happens on the first anastomosis, but not if it happens on the second one!

7. Excessive handling of the vein may lead to thrombosis. To minimize tissue handling, think ahead, know clearly what the plan of action is, and do each step right as you go along so that you do not have to repeat or correct what you have already done. Repetition, hesitation, and correction are each in their own way as traumatic as outright clumsiness.

chapter 9 One-way-up anastomosis

Clinically, small vessel anastomoses often have to be done in spaces more tightly confined and on vessel ends much shorter than those you have seen thus far in the rat. When space and vessel length are very limited, an important constraint comes into effect: it becomes impossible to turn the vessel over to get at the back wall. In preparation for the realities of the clinical world it is important to learn an effective technique for anastomosing vessel ends one-way-up.

To create a situation of deliberately limited access, dissect out only the small length of the femoral artery that lies between Murphy's branch proximally and the epigastric vessel distally. Apply the approximator, taking particular care that the tips of the clamp face toward you. This greatly increases your effective room for maneuver between the clamp jaws. In applying the clamp, include a length of vessel no more than two vessel diameters long. Divide the vessel and prepare the vessel ends. Because the vessel ends are so short, the vessel dilator cannot be used here. For the same reason, only a small quantity of adventitia will present itself for trimming.

Put in the first suture as far away from yourself as possible. The position of this first and only stay stitch is important: you want the whole of the back side of the anastomosis to lie closer to you than the stay stitch. Leave the stitch long and fasten it as directly away from yourself as possible.

The next two or three sutures are made in "upside down" fashion, making two separate passes of the needle, first through the left-hand, then the right-hand tissue edge. Hold the needle as though for any regular suture. Get hold of the near corner of the left-hand vessel end with the left-hand forceps and pull diagonally so that the undersurface of the vessel is brought momentarily into view (Fig. 9-1, *A*). Pass the needle from outside to inside and bring it all the way through. As you get ready for the second pass, make sure that the long tail of the suture, as it emerges from beneath the vessel, is running *toward* you. This is the first of two steps to avoid entanglement. Holding the near corner of the right-hand vessel, pass the needle from inside to outside (Fig. 9-1, *B*).

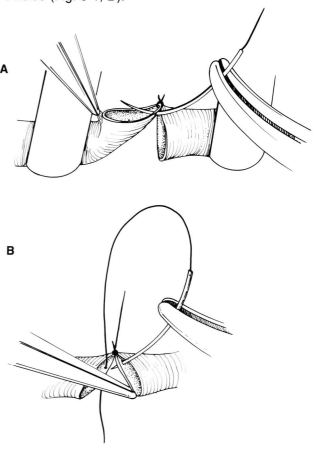

A

B

Fig. 9-1

As you bring the needle tip out, make sure that the needle tip runs past the intraluminal thread on the near side (Fig. 9-2, A) not the far side (Fig. 9-2, B). This is the second step in avoiding a tangle. If the needle tip runs out on the far side of the intraluminal thread a figure-eight entanglement will arise when you tie the knot, with the knot wanting to end up in the lumen.

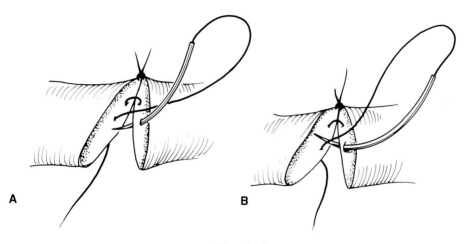

A   B

Fig. 9-2

Tie the knot beneath the vessel and proceed to the next suture. Only the first two or three sutures need to be made in the laborious manner just described. It soon becomes quite easy to flip the underside of the right-hand vessel end into view, as shown in Fig. 9-3.

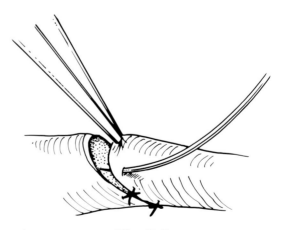

Fig. 9-3

Succeeding stitches can then be placed in simple single-pass fashion. The suturing of the top side of the anastomosis is quite straightforward and does not call for comment.

COMMON PITFALLS

1. Putting the clamps on with the tips facing away from you. This causes your instruments to compete for space with the big end of the clamps, just when you are trying to be dextrous.

2. Putting in the first stitch in the part of the vessel closest to you rather than the part furthest away. This forces you to put in the difficult underside stitches almost blindly.

3. Creating a figure-eight tangle when making the second pass of an underside stitch.

chapter 10 Continuous suture anastomosis

Continuous suturing, in practiced hands, gives results as good as interrupted suturing. However, one wrong stitch or one mistake in thread handling can spoil the whole anastomosis, so practice carefully if you aim to use this technique clinically. Continuous suturing does save time, but only if everything goes just right.

The main hazards in continuous suturing are (1) entanglement while suturing is in progress and (2) purse-string constriction caused by overtightening of the running suture. Entanglement is avoided by starting out with a short thread. Purse-stringing is avoided by the methodical use of two stay sutures placed opposite each other. They not only stretch out the vessel edges but also resist the traction that is put on the thread when you tie the running suture.

Start by cutting your thread short: 3 cm is plenty. Put in the first stitch as close to yourself as possible and fasten it to the near cleat of the suture-holding frame. Cut the unfastened end, leaving it longer than usual, so that another thread can be tied onto it easily (Fig. 10-1).

Put in the second stitch at 180 degrees to the first and tie it with the "short" end quite long. Don't cut either end! Fasten the end without the needle to the far cleat. In doing so, take care to stretch out the vessel edges to their full natural length. With the edges properly stretched out, the distance between

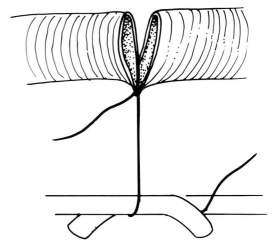

Fig. 10-1

the two stay suture knots is one and a half times the
diameter of the naturally dilated vessel (Fig. 10-2).

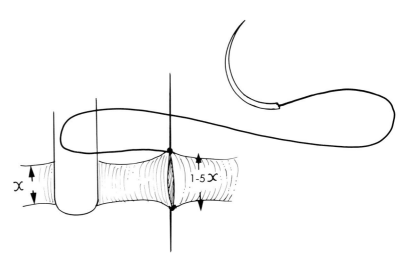

Fig. 10-2

Now you are ready to start the running suture.
Because the front and back edges are equal in
length, there is a greater danger of through-stitching

than usual, so be vigilant in applying the precautions that you have already learned so well. Each side of the anastomosis can be completed with three oblique passes of the needle, or four at most (Fig. 10-3).

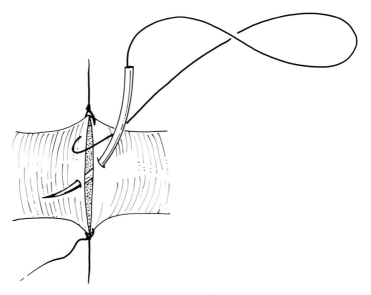

Fig. 10-3

To avoid leakage, the first pass in the row, and also the last, should be as close as possible to the adjacent stay stitch.

With the front side sutured, pull the running stitch tight. This is where purse-stringing would occur, if you didn't have your stay sutures well stretched out and firmly fastened. Provided that the stays are doing their job, the fixed second stay suture, which you pull against as you tighten the running thread, ensures that the tissues can't become bundled up. Now fix the length of the first half by tying the long running thread to the spare end of the first stay suture (Fig. 10-4).

As you tighten this "halfway" knot, be sure that the running thread within the tissues doesn't become

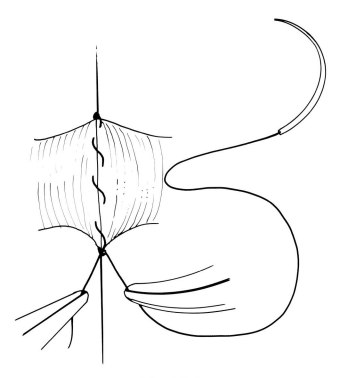

Fig. 10-4

slack. If it does, you will get a leak. Having tied the halfway knot, don't cut either thread.

Pass the needle and thread under the vessel, turn the double clamp over, and you are ready to suture the backside in just the same way as the front (Fig. 10-5).

When you get to the end, unfasten the second stay suture from its cleat and tie the running stitch to it just as you did with the halfway knot. This time the fixed pull of the first stay suture provides the counter traction that prevents overtightening. The appearance of the finished anastomosis should resemble Fig. 10-6.

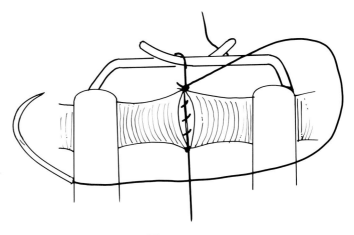

Fig. 10-5

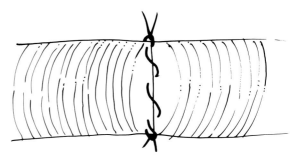

Fig. 10-6

COMMON PITFALLS
1. Starting out with too much thread, thereby producing entanglement.

2. Having the stay sutures too slack or insecurely fastened, so that the full length of the vessel edges is not maintained as the half-way and final knots are tied.

chapter **11** End-to-side anastomosis

Though end-to-side anastomosis comes last in this book, it is not least in importance. Your competence would be most incomplete without the ability to do an end-to-side anastomosis, since in clinical surgery this is often the safest way and sometimes the only way to go. Rat vessels provide a good model of the basics of end-to-side anastomosis. However, there are some aspects of clinical work that you will not encounter on these tiny vessels. These include major inequality of vessel diameter and of vessel wall thickness.

In this exercise the epigastric vein is anastomosed to the common femoral artery to produce an arteriovenous fistula. Interrupted suturing, continuous suturing, and one-way-up suturing will be described.

Before you start, address some reassuring thoughts toward your left hand, since it will be called upon to make a few key moves in this exercise!

PREPARING THE VESSELS

Dissect out the epigastric vein in just the same way as for the vein graft, and dissect out the femoral artery over a sufficient length that you can get a double clamp on it comfortably.

Put a single clamp halfway along the epigastric vein and divide it close to where it emerges from the fat pad. Empty the blood out and dilate the end. Put a double clamp on the artery with the tips facing toward you (Fig. 11-1).

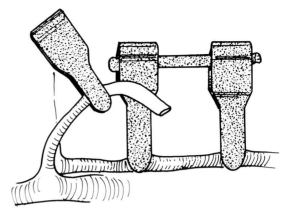

Fig. 11-1

MAKING THE ARTERIOTOMY

In preparation for making the arteriotomy, remove all adventitia thoroughly over an area twice as long and twice as wide as the arteriotomy will be (Fig. 11-2). This is an important step. Adventitia will creep into the arteriotomy with surprising insistence unless you remove it almost all the way around the vessel.

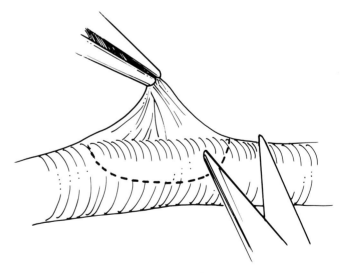

Fig. 11-2

Making the arteriotomy calls for great precision. Two scissor cuts have to be made from opposite directions at 45 degrees to the vessel in such a way that they meet exactly. It is a good idea to practice this maneuver a few times on used-up vessels before doing it for a real anastomosis.

First, right where the middle of the arteriotomy will be, pass one suture transversely through the vessel wall, tie it, and leave it long (Fig. 11-3, A). This gives you a sure way to hold onto the piece you are going to excise.

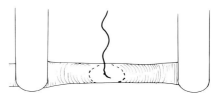

Fig. 11-3, A

Of the two cuts, the second calls for the greatest control, so you will be making it with your right hand. Make the easier first cut with your left hand. With forceps in the right hand, lift straight up on the holding stitch. Hold the adventitia scissors slightly open and at 45 degrees to the vessel (Fig. 11-3, B). The midline of the instrument must lie in the same vertical plane that is made by the vessel and the holding stitch. Correct any rotation of the scissors

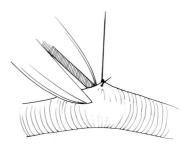

Fig. 11-3, B

about their own long axis to ensure they will make an equal-sided "V" cut in the vessel. Once you are good and ready, cut, going a little less than half way through the vessel.

Wash the blood out of the vessel, change hands, and get ready for the second cut. Aim to make the scissor tips meet exactly at the two ends of the already cut "V" (Fig. 11-3, C). Then go ahead and cut. If your cut stops short, you will have two little

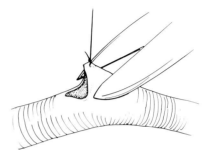

Fig. 11-3, C

bridges of tissue to snip; if it goes too far you will produce a messy "Y" or an even messier "X" where the two cuts cross. You will be lucky if you get the desired result (Fig. 11-3, D) the first time. Keep

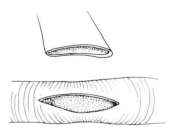

Fig. 11-3, D

practicing, learning as you do so how best to control the exact position of the scissor tips; and learning also at exactly what point, as they close, the tips of your scissors do their last bit of actual cutting.

AVOIDING A TWIST   Before you start suturing, check to see that the vein is not twisted. If you let a twist remain, it will fasten itself on the vessel in an incurable stranglehold at whatever point the vessel has least resistance to twisting.

THE END SUTURES   In suturing, go first to the right hand end of the arteriotomy. Go from outside in through the artery wall first, (Fig. 11-4, *A*) then get repositioned and go from inside out through the vein wall (Fig. 11-4, *B*).

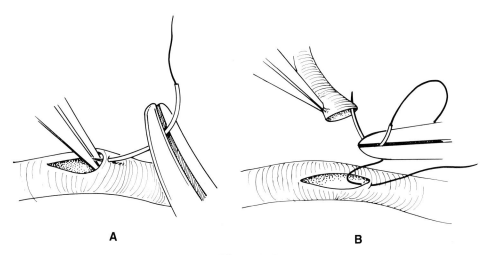

A   B

Fig. 11-4

Doing it this way around maintains a forehand action and avoids the relative difficulty of going from outside in on the loose, free floating vein end. Next put in the left-hand end suture. Since the vein end is still floppy and hard to work on, do this stitch the same way, going from outside in on the artery. This is very much easier to do if you put the needleholder in your left hand (Fig. 11-5, *A* and *B*).

AVOIDING A THROUGH STITCH   In suturing the first of the two sides of the anastomosis, there is a real danger of through-stitching the vein since its front and back edges tend to hang close together. To remove this danger, bring the vein over to expose the far side of the anastomosis and put in one stitch just halfway

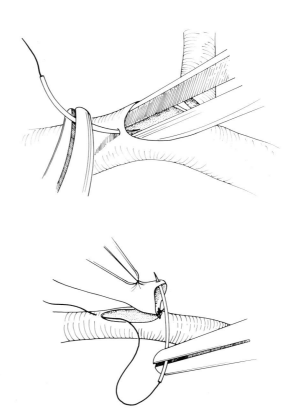

Fig. 11-5

along (Fig. 11-6, *A*). Tie it loosely with only a single half-hitch and leave both ends long. The "V" notch in the back of each artery clamp serves well as a makeshift cleat: pass one suture end over each "V"

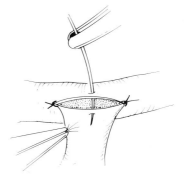

Fig. 11-6, A

notch and give each end a little pull to secure it in place there (Fig. 11-6, *B*). The back edges of your anastomosis will now stay well out of harm's way while you suture the front.

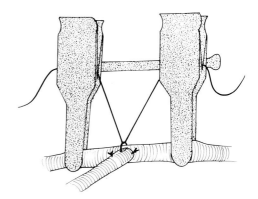

Fig. 11-6, B

THE IMPORTANCE OF RADIAL SUTURING

In all of the suturing that remains, the direction in which your needle passes through the tissue is most important. It should be *radial* to the center of the arteriotomy (Fig 11-7 *A*), not transverse to the main vessel (Fig. 11-7, *B*). This is especially important at

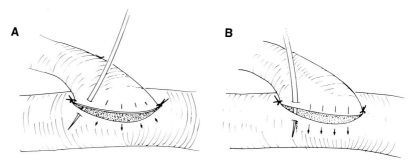

Fig. 11-7

each end of the row. There, a needle passed transversely will produce the same result as a very oblique stitch in end-to-end stitching—one short edge and one long edge. This leads to severe leakage, which is likely to be more persistent in an end-to-side than in an end-to-end anastomosis.

Start suturing the front with a suture at each end, placing it as close as possible to the end suture and passing it radially as shown in Fig. 11-7, *A*. Work from the ends toward the middle, leaving the last few sutures untied until all sutures are in place (Fig. 11-8).

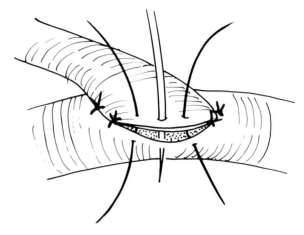

Fig. 11-8

THE BACK SIDE   With the near side completed, turn the vein over toward you to bring the far side back into view. Release and untie the midway stitch and let it hang completely loose. Suture the far side in just the same way as the near side. Take off the proximal clamp for a moment to check for leakage. Leaks at an end-to-side anastomosis tend to go on leaking. If there is any gap in the suture line where leaking blood jumps clear of the vessel, you need to take care of it. If so, reapply the clamp, bombard the anastomosis with Ringer's solution to wash out most of the blood, and put in a partial thickness suture at the offending spot. This is safer than putting in a full-thickness suture blindly, which risks through-stitching.

Finally, take off all the clamps and apply gentle pressure with the fat pad for 2 minutes. Hopefully, the finished result will resemble Fig. 11-9. Patency is indicated by abundant pulsation in the vein and can be checked in case of doubt by an empty and refill test done on the vein.

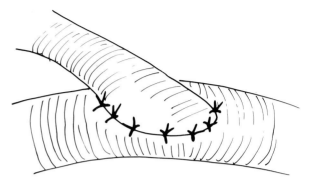

Fig. 11-9

CONTINUOUS SUTURE

Continuous suturing saves time, provided everything goes just right, and is as dependable as interrupted suturing.

Prepare the vessels and make the arteriotomy in just the same way as before. Put in the left-hand end stitch first, leaving both ends long enough that you can tie onto them. Now cut your remaining thread quite short—3 cm is plenty. To have too much thread when you do a running stitch is a big mistake because of the major risk of entanglement that it produces. Put in the right-hand end suture and tie it. To make the continuous row of sutures, you have the choice of passing the needle from vein to artery or from artery to vein throughout the row. Either way works well, but one is always less awkward than the other in terms of instrument and hand position—especially when you get to the end of the row. Look ahead before you start stitching and see which suturing direction will become easiest for you at the end of the row; take that direction from the start. Pass each individual suture of the row in the same radial direction as you would in interrupted suturing (Fig. 11-10).

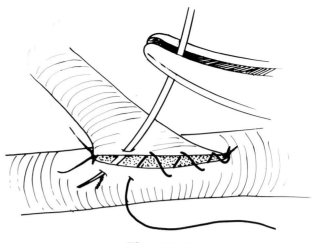

Fig. 11-10

Be sure to get the next-to-the-end sutures as close as possible to the end sutures. Do not pull the running suture tight at all as you go along or you will end up suturing blindly. Once you have the row completed, tighten up the running thread in two stages. First, go along the row from right to left, pulling each loop semitight. Then take the short, cut end of the starting knot in your right-hand forceps and the long end of the thread in your left-hand forceps. Pull on the long end until the running stitch in the tissues becomes almost straight (Fig. 11-11).

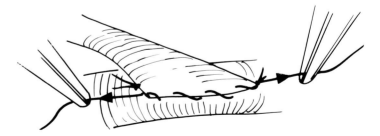

Fig. 11-11

The countertraction you exert while doing this with the right-hand forceps is most important. It prevents excessive strain from falling on the tissues and, more importantly, it prevents overtightening, which can readily lead to purse string constriction.

With the thread tightened, tie the long end to one end of the initial left-hand stitch. Beware of overtightening! As you make the knot, watch to be sure the running thread comes just as tight as you made it with your two-handed pull but not a fraction tighter. Cut both ends short, turn the vein over, and suture the far side in exactly the same way as the near side. To finish, tie the second running thread to the other short end of the initial left hand knot.

ONE-WAY-UP SUTURING

Until now you have enjoyed the comfort and convenience of having an abundant length of side vessel to work with. This has enabled you to turn the vein over from one side of the artery to the other, making the far side just as accessible and easy as the near side. In real life you cannot always get this much side vessel to work with. Often the side vessel only just reaches the arteriotomy. When this is so you should not hesitate to do the anastomosis one-way-up, suturing the far side from within the vessel.

To give yourself a short vein situation, prepare the vessels as before but bring the vein around the bar of the clamp so that it cannot be swung around freely (Fig. 11-12).

Put in the first suture on the left, and begin the running suture as you did before. Now hold the needle so that the point is toward you, take it round behind the right-hand end suture, and pass it from outside in through the artery close to the end stitch (Fig. 11-13, A). Make this blind half-stitch cautiously: if you see that the needle is starting to come through at a bad spot, back off and correct yourself. Having passed the needle, pull all the thread through and you are ready to do the inside-out suturing of the

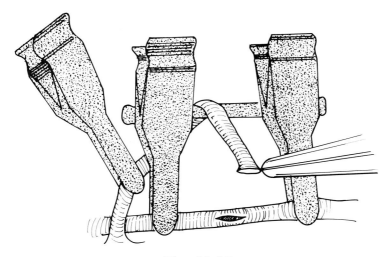

Fig. 11-12

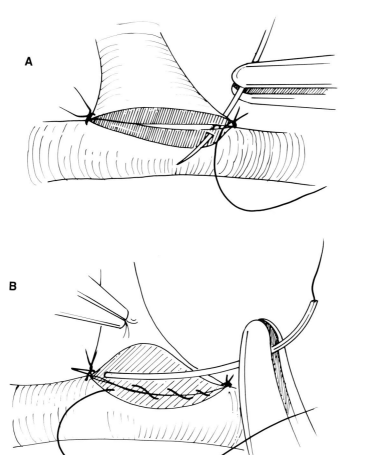

Fig. 11-13

back wall, which is entirely straightforward. When you get to the end, make an exit half-stitch through the vein and tie on to one end of the left-hand end stitch as before (Fig. 11-13, *B*). Suturing the front side presents no problem at all.

COMMON PITFALLS

1. Not removing adventitia widely and thoroughly at the site of the arteriotomy.

2. Making an untidy arteriotomy, especially where the two cuts meet.

3. Making the arteriotomy too large—profuse leakage results.

4. Having the side vessel twisted at the outset.

5. Through-stitching the side vessel edges.

6. Passing the needle in the wrong direction, straight across the artery rather than radial to the center of the arteriotomy.

7. Leaving a gap between an end stitch and its neighbor.

In continuous suturing

1. Getting entangled with an excessive length of thread.

2. Overtightening as the running stitch is tied, leading to purse-string constriction.

3. In short-side-vessel situations, struggling to get at the inaccessible back edges from outside rather than calmly suturing back edges from inside.

Always remember that in microvascular surgery, to struggle is to invite disaster!

Appendix

All the items described in Chapter 1, except the most everyday ones, are listed below, together with catalog number and approximate 1988 price. Suppliers and addresses are on the following page. When dealing directly with the sales departments of large companies, either have ready an official purchase order from your institution and be able to quote its serial number, or else ask for the goods to be shipped COD.

SUPPLIES

Equipment	Supplier	Catalog no.	Approximate price (in dollars)
Straight jeweler's forceps	S&T	ST-JFL 3	16.00
Angled jeweler's forceps	S&T	ST-JFAL 3	30.00
Needleholder	S&T	ST-BL-13	160.00
Vessel dilator	S&T	ST-D5aZ	37.00
Scissors, dissecting	S&T	ST-SDC-11	115.00
Scissors, adventitia	S&T	ST-SAS-11	115.00
Vessel clamps, 11 mm double approximator with suture-holding frame	S&T	ST-ABB-2V	110.00
Vessel clamps, 8 mm double approximator without suture-holding frame	S&T	ST-ABB-11V	70.00
Vessel clamps, 8 mm single, 1 pair	S&T	ST-B-1V	17.00
Instrument case	S&T	ST-ICF-1020	115.00

Bipolar coagulator unit	Codman	80-1114	895
Bipolar forceps and cord	Weck	392000	42
Microsuture, 10/0 nylon, 100 micron flat-bodied taper point needle, in unsterile lab packs	Ethicon	2889 (pack of 72 sutures)	563
Microsuture, 10/0 nylon, 75 micron flat-bodied taper point needle, in unsterile lab packs	Ethicon	2888 (pack of 72 sutures)	762
Demagnetizer	Assi	AD-19-202	52
Microscope transport cart	Harper Truck	2456-69	204
Clippers	Oster	A5	129
Fine hair cutter for clippers	Oster	A5	20
Instrument repair pliers (Lindstrom)	Casker Co.	PL 7490	35
Emery paper, 4/0	S&T	ST-PP4	5
Blue polyethylene background material	Oates Flap	1 square yard	2

SUPPLIERS

Assi (Accurate Surgical and
Scientific Instruments Corporation)
300 Shames Drive
Westbury, New York 11590   800-645-3569

Casker Company
2121 Spring Grove Avenue
Cincinnati, Ohio 45214   800-847-4188

Codman & Shurtlett, Inc.
Pacella Park Drive
Randolph, Massachusetts 02368   617-961-2300

Harper Trucks, Inc.
P.O. Box 12330
Wichita, Kansas 67277   316-942-1381

Oates Flap Company
329 East Market Street
Louisville, Kentucky 40202   800-431-4766

Oster Corporation
5055 North Lydell
Milwaukee, Wisconsin 53217   414-332-8300

S&T Microlab AG
Zollstrasse 91
CH-8212 Neuhausen am Rheinfall
Switzerland   (011-31) 53-27406

Edward Weck & Company
P.O. Box 12600
Research Triangle Park,
North Carolina 27709   800-334-8511

INDEX

131

Venous pressure, raising, 96
Vessel clamps, 7-8
Vessel dilator, 6
Vessels; *see* Artery; Veins
Visual contrast, background material for, 13

W

Workbench, 12
Wriggling
  common femoral artery, 73

Wriggling—cont'd
  false, 73
Writing position for hands, 22-24

X

Xylocaine; *see* Lidocaine

Z

Zeiss microscope, 11